Application of Nursing Theories

Application of Nursing Theories

Ajesh Kumar TK MSc (N)
Lecturer
College of Nursing
All India Institute of Medical Sciences
New Delhi, India

Soumya Chandran MSc (N)
Nursing Officer
All India Institute of Medical Sciences
New Delhi, India

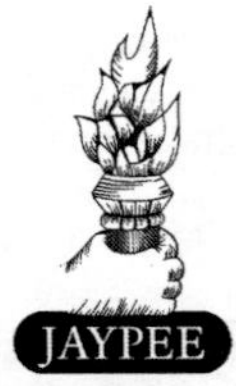

JAYPEE BROTHERS MEDICAL PUBLISHERS
The Health Sciences Publisher
New Delhi | London

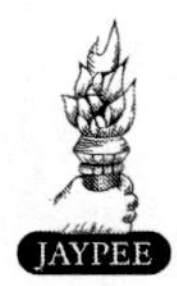

Jaypee Brothers Medical Publishers (P) Ltd

Headquarters
EMCA House
23/23-B, Ansari Road, Daryaganj
New Delhi - 110 002, India
Landline: +91-11-23272143, +91-11-23272703
+91-11-23282021, +91-11-23245672
E-mail: jaypee@jaypeebrothers.com

Corporate Office
4838/24, Ansari Road, Daryaganj
New Delhi - 110 002, India
Phone: +91-11-43574357
Fax: +91-11-43574314
E-mail: jaypee@jaypeebrothers.com

Overseas Office
J.P. Medical Ltd
83 Victoria Street, London
SW1H 0HW (UK)
Phone: +44 20 3170 8910
E-mail: info@jpmedpub.com

EU GPSR Authorised Representative
Logos Europe, 9 rue Nicolas Poussin
17000, La Rochelle, France
Phone: +33 (0) 6 67 93 73 78
E-mail: contact@logoseurope.eu

Website: www.jaypeebrothers.com
Website: www.jaypeedigital.com

Inquiries for bulk sales may be solicited at: jaypee@jaypeebrothers.com

Application of Nursing Theories

First Edition: 2017, Reprint: 2026

ISBN: 978-93-86150-63-9

Printed at: Samrat Offset Pvt. Ltd.

Preface

With praises to our Lord, the Giver of life from Whom all good things come, we introduce you to *Application of Nursing Theories* with immense sense of gratitude. It is undoubtedly true that nursing has undergone numerous changes from the past few decades. One of these trends is to shift towards theory-based nursing care. Nursing theories describe and relate to the different aspects of practice and give as a framework for systemizing the nursing practice. These theories guide us about what questions to ask, what to observe, how to evaluate our practice and how to advance in the field. We honor the works of eminent nursing theorists whose contribution have catalyzed this shift.

The main objective of writing this book is to simplify the abstract concepts of nursing theories and accelerate the application of these theories into nursing practice, nursing education and nursing research thereby improving the quality of nursing care.

This book focuses on the concepts of various nursing theories and application of these theories into nursing with a case scenario. This book is divided into three units. *Unit I: Introduction to Nursing Theories* illustrates the terminologies, evolution and types of nursing theories and how it can be used in nursing practice. *Unit II: Grand Nursing Theories* provides illustration of fourteen nursing grand theories along with its application. Finally, *Unit III: Middle-Range Nursing Theories* focuses on the sixteen middle-range nursing theories. Each chapter covers a detailed description of a theory categorized under biography of the author, assumptions, major concepts, metaparadigm in nursing, application into nursing education, practice and research, nursing process, case scenario and critique of the theory. We hope that this book will prove beneficial for the nursing scholars and nurses alike.

Ajesh Kumar TK
Soumya Chandran

Acknowledgments

I wish to express my gratitude to the Almighty Who has been immensely blessing me throughout this work.

Thank you to the following individuals without their contributions and support, this book would not have been possible:

My wife Anila, our son, Karthik, my parents, brothers, sisters-in-law, nieces, nephews and family members of my in-laws for being in my life.

My Teachers especially Dr Theresa Mathias who remains my mentor, motivator and well-wisher.

The supportive colleagues of Maharishi Markandeshwar College of Nursing, Mullana, Ambala, Haryana, India and College of Nursing, All India Institute of Medical Sciences, New Delhi, India particularly Dr Jyoti Sarin and Dr Manju Vatsa.

My friends noticeably Sanoob Devasia, Dr Achla Dagdu Gaikwad, Sembian N, Manu KJ, Jomin Jose, Riji Geevarghese, Anju R Pillai, Sooraj K John, Rashmi Panchal, Majari Rana, Kuldeep Kaur Sandhar, Yogesh Kumar, Malarkodi, Rosmin George, Nirmaljeet Kaur, Dr Poonam Sheoran, Vinay Kumari, Srinivasan P, Uma Deaver, for constant motivation and support which gives me strength and comfort.

I would like to thank Ms Ruby Sharma, Project Manager and all other staff members of Jaypee Brothers Medical Publishers, New Delhi for their continuous support for making this book.

My loving Students who really encouraged me to write this book to simplify nursing theories.

Finally, I beg forgiveness to all those who have been with me during this project and whose names I have failed to mention.

Ajesh Kumar TK

Acknowledgments

I wish to personally thank the following for their contributions to my inspiration and knowledge and other help in creating this book.

With utmost humility I would like to praise and thank Almighty God, the merciful and compassionate Who bestowed me with the health, sense and courage to go through crucial time.

This book is a result of many helping hands and without their support and encouragement, it would not have been possible to complete a work of this magnitude.

Most importantly, none of this would have been possible without the love, support and patience of my family. I would like to express my heartfelt gratitude to my husband, Sajimon and our son, Ishan, daughter Idika, parents and in-laws for all their help and support.

This manuscript would never have taken shape without the inspiration and support of my teachers, friends and colleagues. So I express my gratitude and love towards them.

I would like to express my grateful thanks to all the staff members of Jaypee Brothers Medical Publishers, New Delhi for their valuable support for making this book.

Last but not the least, let me express my appreciation to all those who have inspired me directly or indirectly to complete this book.

Soumya Chandran

Contents

UNIT I

INTRODUCTION TO NURSING THEORIES

UNIT II

GRAND NURSING THEORIES

UNIT III

MIDDLE-RANGE NURSING THEORIES

Unit I

INTRODUCTION TO NURSING THEORIES

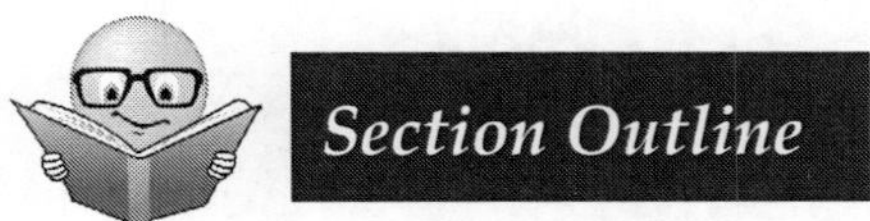

Introduction to Nursing Theories

Nursing has undergone exceptional accomplishment in the last three decades. It has moved from direct patient care towards theory based practice which made the modern nursing more significant and consequential to make nursing as an ordered profession. Theories are an explanation of the relationship between the phenomena. Theory is defined as a set of concepts, definitions, relationships, and assumptions that project a systematic view of a phenomenon. Nursing phenomena are the central elements of nursing domain help the person, nurse and environment. Nursing theories describes and relates the different aspects of practice and give as a framework for systemizing the nursing practice. This theories guide us in what questions to ask, what to observe, how to evaluate our practice and how to advance the field.

Terminologies Related to Nursing Theories

Concepts: Ideas and notions used to describe phenomena.

Definitions: Express the meaning of concepts.

Assumptions: These are the explanation of concepts.

Phenomenon: A situation or a reality that can be measurable or observable.

Construct: It is those phenomena which cannot be testable.

Proposition: Narrates the link between concepts.

Processes: The series of actions, changes which are proposed to bring about a desired result.

Conceptual framework: A group of concepts that are defined and scientifically ordered to give a focus, a justification, and an instrument for the integration and understanding of information.

A *paradigm* is a model that explains the linkages of science, philosophy, and theory accepted and applied by the discipline.

Nursing paradigms are mold employed to demonstrate an association among the available nursing theories. The main focus of nursing theories into four major concepts—Person/Client, Health, Environment and Nursing.

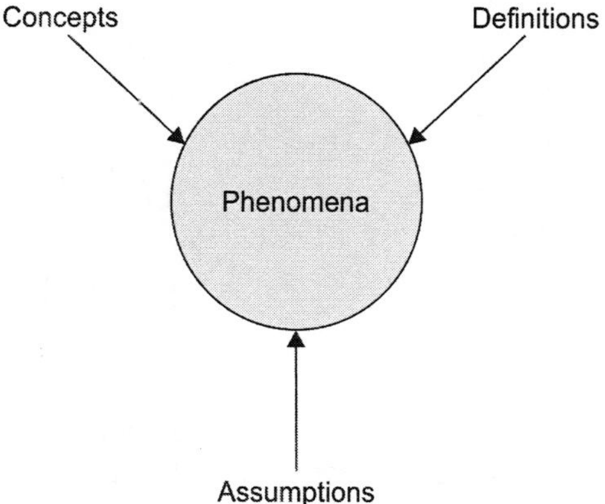

Fig. I.1: Components of nursing theories

METAPARADIGM IN NURSING

Nursing paradigms are mold employed to demonstrate an association among the available nursing theories. These given concepts vary in accordance to the experiences and views of different nursing theorists. These four major paradigms in nursing, i.e. Person/Client, Health, Environment and Nursing.

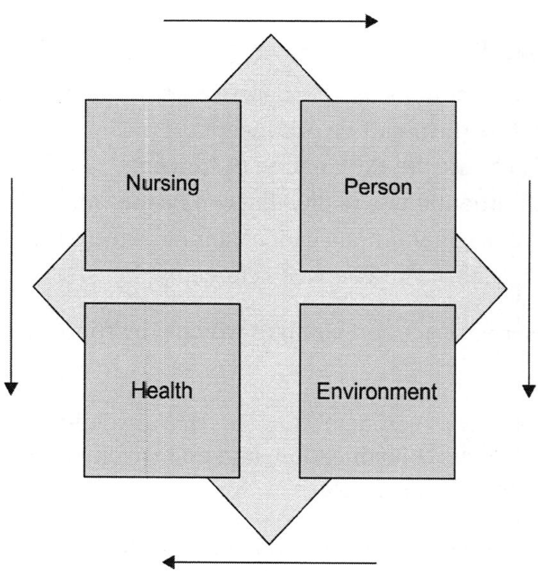

Fig. I.2: Major paradigms in nursing

Person

The concept of person was established in ANAs definition is as individual, families, communities and population'. They are the participator in nursing. Persons have specific need and priorities nurse goals is to meet these needs thus leads to optimal health.

Environment

Environment here could be a patient's significant others, physical surrounding as well as local or economic conditions that can be linked to the person's life and health status. Nursing can then help the individual modify the environment through the practices given.

Health

Health is a dynamic state, a combination of wellness and illness. Wellness, in this view, is the lived experience of congruence between one's possibilities and one's realities and is based on caring and feeling cared for.

Nursing

American Nurses Association (2012) defines nursing as—'the protection, promotion and optimization of health and abilities, prevention of illness and injury, alleviation of suffering through the nursing diagnosis and treatment of human response; and advocacy in the care individual, families, communities and population.

TYPES OF NURSING THEORY

Theories of nursing have been classified into different categories by the many authors.

Grand Nursing theories: This type of theory is considered as the most conceptual among all other theory. It is very extensive and multifarious. It is always proposing things which can be testable. Some of the examples of grand Nursing theories are as following:

- Faye Abdellah - **21 Typology Nursing Problems**
- Lydia Hall - Core, Care and Cure Circles
- Virginia Henderson - **14 Components of Basic Nursing Care**
- Dorothy Johnson - Behavioral System Model
- Imogene King - Open Systems Theory
- Levine - Conservation Model
- Betty Neuman - Systems Theory
- Florence Nightingale - Environmental Theory
- Dorothea Orem - Self-Care Deficit Theory
- Martha Rogers - **The Science of Unitary Human Beings**
- Callista Roy - Adaptation Theory
- Joyce Travelbee - Human to Human Relationship Model

- Jean Watson - Theory of Caring
- Ernestine Wiedenbach - Prescriptive theory—A situation producing theory.

Middle-range Nursing theories: These theories are the least abstract among all other theory. It address precise observable fact and replicate practice. These theories are able to reach a specific population, given place or time with the process usually beginning at a simple, single descriptor concept. It is very constructive for nursing research and practice:

- Adam Evelyn **- Conceptual Model for Nursing**
- Dr Bennett Mary - PNI Nursing Theory
- Carr JM - Nursing Theory of Vigilance
- Dr Kolcaba K - The Comfort Theory
- Larrabee J - Quality of Nursing Care
- Leininger M - Transcultural Nursing
- Rozzano Locsin - Advancing Technology, Caring and Nursing
- Ida Jean Orlando - The Deliberative Nursing Process
- Dr Nola J Pender **- Health Promotion Model**
- Hildegard E Peplau - Interpersonal Relations
- Larry D Purnell **- Purnell's Model for Cultural Competence**
- Barbara Resnick **- Middle Range Nursing Theory of Self-efficacy**
- Reva Rubin **- Theory of Maternal Identity**
- Cornelia Ruland **- End of Life Care**
- Kristen M Swanson - Theory of Caring.

Descriptive Nursing Theories: It is first level of theory development and this type of theory describes a phenomena, event or a situation. These are produced and tested by descriptive research. The main two types of descriptive theory are *factors isolating and category formulating.* Factor isolating explains the characteristics and dimensions of an event. Category formulating narrates the types of relationship between one event to the other event. These theories are needed when nothing is known about particular phenomena. This theory explains the relationship and predict the nursing phenomena.

Prescriptive Nursing Theories: This theory tells us nursing intervention and foresee their effect on the patient. It includes all suggestion to that need to change or modify, and foresee the effect of those particular nursing interventions. It expresses certain components in nursing such as client basic life process, interaction with the environment and its effect on the wellness of the client.

 HISTORICAL DEVELOPMENT OF NURSING THEORIES

The evolution of the nursing theories is marked by several milestones that have been identified by conducting thorough reviews on the various sources from 1950 to 2000.

From Florence Nightingale to Development of Nursing Research

- Florence nightingale (1860), by manipulating the patient environment we could best influence our patient health. Proper light, fresh air, hygienic conditions, absence of noise among the others factors that would allow body to right itself and heal.
- The key landmark before 1955 was the establishment of Nursing Research Journal for reporting the researches and scientific evidences for nursing by the nurses.

Origin of Nursing Theory from 1955 to 1960

- Peplau (1952), developed the first expressed concept in nursing on interpersonal relationship between the nurse and patient are the key factor in providing best nursing care.
- Subsequently others theories was developed in the 1960s by using the Peplau's ideas.
- Virginia Henderson set up 14 components of Basic Nursing Care in 1955.
- Dorethea Orem's ideas were first published in Guidelines for Developing Curricula for the Education of Practical Nurses in 1959.
- Faye abdellah, et al. in 1960 – Nursing as a comprehensive service to meet patient's need thereby increases or restores self-help ability by Using 21 problems to guide nursing care.

Theory: A National Goal for Nursing: 1961 to 1965

- Attention focused on to the patient as a set of need and nursing as a set of unique functions.
- Establishment of another journal, i.e. nursing sciences.

1966–1970: Theory of Development a Real Goal for Academics

- Nursing theories started to get recognition and found that theses are very essential for the practice.
- Definition of and goal of nursing theories formulated.
- Dorothy Johnson 1968—describes the patient's adjustment with the stress and how theses stress will affect the health of an individual. Nursing action was mainly focused to reduce the stress which are affecting the patients.
- The metatheorists Ellis (1968), Widenbach Dickoff (1968) and James (1968) questioned about what types of theories nurses has to develop and the content need to include in nursing theories.
- *Rogers, Martha Elizabeth 1970:* Nursing interventions should be noninvasive activities, such as therapeutic touch, humor, guided imagery, meditation which are mainly for promoting the health of a patients. She considered person as a Unitary Human Being.

1971–1975: Theory Syntax

- Mainly focus was on the theory development and the components for theory.
- Metatheorist continued to question the meaning of nursing theory, components, how to analyze and evaluate the theories.
- *Dorothea Orem 1971:* Nursing interventions was mainly focusing on assisting or providing self-care to the patients. This assistance will leads to promotion of health and adjustments with the effect of illness.
- *Imogene King 1971:* She was mainly focusing on the interaction between the nurse and patient, patient's involvement in decision-making or participation in care. During the interaction process they mutually exchange the information, set goals and try to achieve those goals.
- *Betty Neuman 1972:* This theory is mainly focusing on the stresser's actual or potential response of patients and by application of primary, secondary, territory interventions in order to tackle this stressors.
- National league for nursing recognized the theory and a curriculum based on the theory as mandatory requirement for accreditation of nursing school.
- This landmark in the history of nursing history leads to more development and uses of nursing theories.

1976–1980: The Time to Replicate

- Many of the nurse theorist were invited by the various institutions for their lectures, discussion.
- Another Journal Advances in Nursing was established and its main focus was theory development, analysis and evaluation of it.
- Sr Callista Roy 1979—describes person as an adaptive system and the main responses of the patients can be adaptive or ineffective. The nursing action focuses on promoting the adaptive responses.
- The connection between the research and theory were addressed. The more ways were identified to close the gap between the research and practice of theory.
- Jean Watson 1979—theory of caring explains caring as creative factors that results in the fulfillment of human needs and ultimately it promotes the positive health of an individual or family. The use of caring is the central key for nursing practice.

1981–1985: Nursing Theories Revitalization

- Nursing theories started to get acceptances in the various countries.
- Theories becomes a tool to solve the problems in nursing practice as well as a guide for the practice.
- New York University started nursing program on advanced theoretical nursing and also given the a lucid illustration of how a nursing school can use nursing theory.

1986–1990: Evolution from Matatheory to Development of Concepts

- Ongoing debates and discussion on nursing theories leads to an increase in concept development and evaluation of it.
- It also leads to recognize breach between theory and practice.
- Successful analyses were carried out on the main nursing concept such as environment, person health.

1991–1995: Era of a Situation Specific Theories

Numerous middle range theories were evolved in this period which mainly addressed a specific nursing practice and reflection on nursing practice.

1996–2000: Evidence Means Research

- Started to scrutinize the various concepts and theories. In addition main focus was on recognizing the similarities and differences of these theories on the basis of evidences.
- Evidences started to get appreciation globally and the period of evidenced based practice evolved.

2001–2005: Bridging the Theory and Practices

Mainly focused on the multiplicity in the theory development and the various ways to apply or utilize theoretical concepts into practice.

CRITIQUE OF NURSING THEORY

It is the evaluation of a theory and it can be done by analyzing the five main components, i.e. *simplicity, clarity, generality, empirical precision* and *derivable consequences* of a theory.

Simplicity is a highly valid point and it means how easy the theory and level of difficulty in the concepts.

Clarity means the uniformity in the words uses in the theory, clearly stated concepts, clear relationship between the each concept and easy to understand.

Generality is the scope of application of the theory. A theory must have a broad scope and it should not be constrained within the specific time or situation.

Empirical precision is the testability and usefulness of a theory. For testing the theory of concepts should be measurable or observable.

Derivable consequences of a theory indicate the usefulness and importance of it. According to Chinn and Kramer a theory must be evaluated on the bases of social, political and environmental consequences also. They suggested that those theories are not socially responsible that cannot be used in nursing.

CONCLUSION

All nursing theories a definite nursing action which we can make our clients level of wellness. We all of us imploy nursing theory in all steps of the nursing process, which include assessment, planning, implementing, and evaluating nursing action.

Unit II

GRAND NURSING THEORIES

Section Outline

1. Florence Nightingale: Environmental Adaptation Theory
2. Faye Abdellah: Twenty-one Typology Nursing Problems
3. Lydia Eloise Hall: Core, Care and Cure Circles
4. Virginia Henderson: Fourteen Components of Basic Nursing Care
5. Dorothy E Johnson: Behavioral System Model
6. Imogene King: Theory of Goal Attainment
7. Myra Levine: Conservation Model
8. Betty Neuman: Systems Theory
9. Dorothea Orem: Self-Care Deficit Theory
10. Martha Rogers: The Science of Unitary Human Beings
11. Callista Roy: Adaptation Theory
12. Joyce Travelbee: Human to Human Relationship Model
13. Jean Watson: Theory of Caring
14. Ernestine Wiedenbach: Prescriptive Theory—A Situation Producing Theory

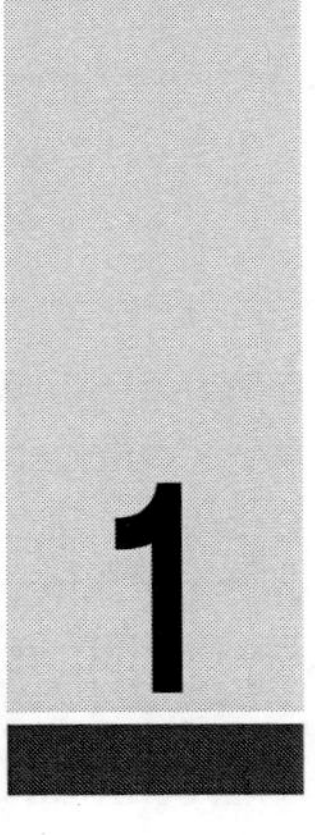

1 Florence Nightingale: Environmental Adaptation Theory

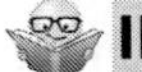 INTRODUCTION

The impact of environment on our health where we live is not simply shrugged off. This is the main concept of the Nightingales' assumption. It is the fundamental responsibility of every nurse to maintain a conducive hospital atmosphere by providing pure water, air, light and maintaining proper cleanliness and efficient drainage system.

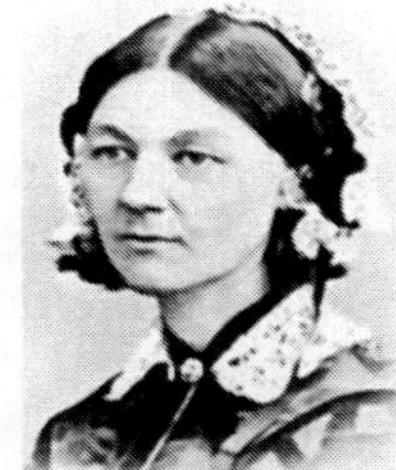

Florence Nightingale

Biography

- She was born in 1820 in Florence, Italy—the city was named after her.
- In the very young age, she was very inquisitive and on the go in the humanitarian works especially for ill and poor people nearby her family.
- In the mid teen years she realized her interest on nursing as career perspective. Despite of nightingales' parents' objection towards her ambition, she was determined to pursue her wish.
- In 1844, Nightingale enrolled as a nursing student at the Lutheran Hospital of Pastor Fliedner in Kaiserswerth, Germany.
- After training, she went to London and worked as nurse in Middlesex hospital for sick governesses in 1850. Hospital authorities were impressed by her work and gave promotion to the post of superintendant within one year.
- During the cholera outbreak in London she worked extensively in improving the sanitary condition owing to a significant decrease in Cholera associated mortality rate.
- In 1854, the aftermath of the Crimean War led to dwindling of British soldiers, the poor sanitation facilities at the war site hospitals accelerated this mortality rate.
- The Secretary of War Sidney Herbert requested Nightingale to arrange a team and move to Crimea for treating wounded soldiers.
- She immediately followed his order and formed that the condition of the battlefield was worst than she expected.
- She realized that poor environmental and scarcity of basic supplies as the main catalyst for hike in the mortality rate and worked on improvement in these areas.

- Surprisingly, her relentless efforts produced a drastic decline in mortality rate among soldiers. For this persistent work she received many accolades and named as 'Lady with the Lamp.'
- In 1857, she wrote the first book on nursing 'Notes on Nursing' after analyzing the condition of Crimean War and even today which is considered as cornerstone for the nursing curriculum.
- Nightingale utilized the prize money for her work from British Government to build Nightingale Training School for Nurses in St Thomas Hospital at London in 1960.
- Many young both poor and wealthy enrolled in her nursing school and became successful nurses. One of the notable among them is Lind Richard.
- Nightingale returned to Scutari and spent rest of her life there in assisting various hospitals and nursing institutes to implement her environmental model to promote patient care.

Assumptions

- The main components which are vital for a health of houses are pure air, pure water, efficient drainage, cleanliness and light.
- Nursing is an art and a science.
- Nursing encompasses caring the patient through maintaining a healthy environment which is conducive for healing.
- Nurses need to undergo certain special training in order to practice nursing.
- Nursing profession is entirely different from physicians.'

Concepts

Environmental Adaptation Model

The focus of nursing is to change the patient's environment to maintain his or her health. The environment can be physical, psychological and social.

Components of a Healthful Environment

- *Health of houses:* Concentrates on the five essentials of pure air, pure water, efficient drainage, cleanliness, and light, 'without these, no house can be healthy'
- *Ventilation and Warming:* It is very indispensable to create frequent flow of air in patient's room in order to keep them healthy. Nightingale believed that stagnant air in the patient room can deteriorate the patient health. It is also essential to keep the optimum room temperature.
- *Light:* Light has tangible effects to the body. Hence the nurses should include direct exposure to sunlight in their interventions.
- *Cleanliness:* She considered that poor living condition and personal hygiene are the main source of infection. Nursing interventions pertains

to this aspects are proper treatment of body secretions and sewage, bathing, clean cloths and handwashing.

- *Nutrition:* Nightingale noted that people interest towards food is unique and varies at different times of the day. She also mentioned the need for small and frequent meals instead of heavy one time food.
- *Variety:* Changes in the patient room are very essential to keep the patient active and fresh. This can be done by changing the flower pot or engravings of patient room.
- *Bed and Bedding:* The bed should be positioned near the window so that patient could see out of the window. She also asserted the importance of changing the beddings frequently.
- *Chattering Hopes and Advices:* False reassurance on the illness should be avoided and sick person need to hear the good news which will assist him to be healthier.

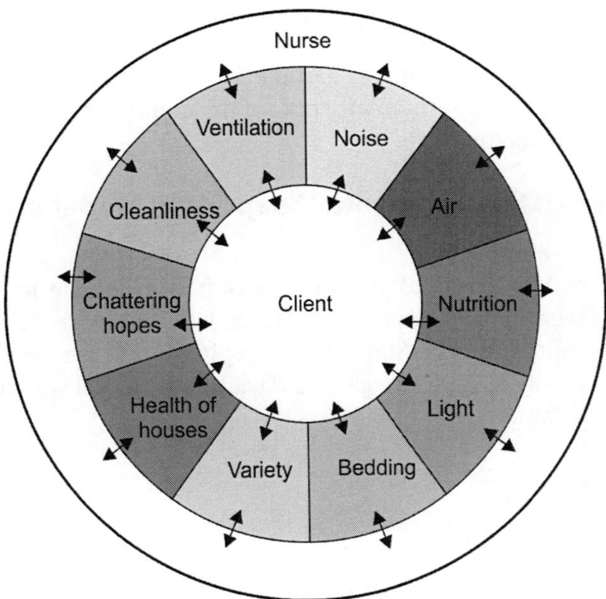

Fig. 1.1: Conceptual frame work based on environmental adaptation model

METAPARADIGM IN NURSING

Person: Patient is the passive receiver of nursing care. Human beings are in constant interaction with the environment and any minute changes in the surrounding can affect them.

Environment: The external conditions which have direct influence on patient. When the environment is in disequilibrium the patient need to use energy in order to adjust with it.

Health: It is not properly defined by Nightingale. She believed that health can be maintained by prevention of illness through environmental modification.

Nursing: According to Nightingale '*What nursing has to do... is to put the patient in the best condition for nature to act upon him*'. A nurse ensures proper water, air, light and maintaining proper cleanliness and efficient drainage system for environment to act on patient.

Application of Environmental Adaptation Model

Nursing Practice: The entire nursing field is highly influenced by Nightingale theory. Manipulation of environment remains the foundation of contemporary nursing.

Nursing Education: Environmental adaptation is the fundamental guide for the nursing curriculum across the globe. She asserted that nursing school should be sovereign from the hospital.

Nursing Research: Nightingale found many basis for scientific enquiry in nursing. Nonetheless, her theory is short of the complexity and testability of the modern nursing theories.

Application of Environmental Adaptation Model in Nursing Process

Case Scenario: Mrs Y age 48 years has admitted in female medical ward, diagnosis of fever. She had complaints of fever with headache, chills, diarrhea, rigor malaise and anorexia. She was in hospital for 5 days. Her laboratory report shows plenty of WBCs in urine and waiting for blood and urine culture report, chest X-ray shown normal.

Assessment

Physical Environment

- Presence of enough window and proper ventilation.
- Presence of fowl smelly dumping site outside the window.
- Having proper light but no direct sun light to the bed.
- Well facility for hot water twice a day but without purification.
- Ward toilet drainage system is good but presence of food particles and dust in the pan and around the pan.
- Room environment is clean and ward is swiped frequently.
- Presence of water leakage around the sink.
- Having only one piece of biscuits with milk, one full cup of dhal and 1 glass of plain water during 6 hours period.
- Bed is clean and tidy but presence of food particles and cover of medicines, pieces of papers and dust inside the locker.
- Cool room temperature.

- Patient is covered with two blankets but still feeling cold.
- Hospital is located centrally near to the main city so there is noise of horn, loudspeakers.

Psychological Environment

- Mrs has never been admitted in hospital before.
- Feeling uncomfortable and have trouble in sleep.
- She felt that noise because of presence of nursing station near to her bed.
- She is very active woman and feels her time is wasted since the admission.

Social Environment

- Patient told that her home environment is clean.
- They use to drink boiling water.
- Her room is small but with enough ventilation and sunlight.
- No history of illness like her in the family or neighborhood.

Nursing Diagnosis

- Risk for infection related to unsafe drinking water, dust from locker, dirt from sink and outside of the room.
- Risk for injury related wet floor.
- Altered nutrition less than body requirement related to inadequate intake of food.
- Altered comfort measures related to strange, noisy and cold environment.

Goal

- Mrs Y will be free from infection during hospital stay as evidence by normal WBCs range.
- Client will be free from injury as evidence by not slip on the floor.
- Client's nutrition level will be maintained as evidence by constant weight till hospitalization.
- Client will feel comfortable as evidence by absence of noise near to the nursing station and increase room temperature.

Intervention

- Provided purified and boiling water for drinking according to patient demand.
- Cleaned the locker routinely and keep all medicines in small paper box or medicine bag.
- Informed to the incharge for maintenance of sink, waste disposal.
- Kept the surrounding clean.
- Provided adequate diet by encouraging small frequent and nutritious feeding.
- Maintained temperature by proper dress up and provide extra blanket.
- Adhered to the biomedical waste management protocol

- Kept the patient in calm and comfortable position and avoid unnecessary stimulation, noise.
- Provided sufficient support and advice related to disease process, diet therapy.

Evaluation

- She told that she is getting boiled and purified water.
- She said that she has no vomiting and loose motion.
- She has gained a weight and no feeling of weakness and increased appetite.
- Locker is cleaned and no presence of dust around the sink.

Critique

Clarity and Simplicity: The concepts in the environmental adaptation model areas very clear and followed a logical sequence.

Generality: This theory is having a wide horizon of application. Some of the concepts can be easily adapt into the every spheres of nursing practice ranges from hospital to a vast community. Nevertheless, ventilation is not always been bliss for the patients, the contaminated air can infect an open wound or a burned skin.

Empirical Precision: Nightingale theory lacks the complexity and testability of the modern nursing theories.

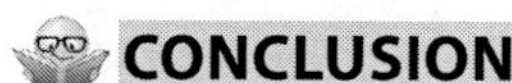

CONCLUSION

Florence Nightingale developed the first model of nursing care that is grounded in the belief that alteration of the environment will prevent disease. Hence it is the onus of every nurse to maintain a smoothening environment health promotion of patients and themselves.

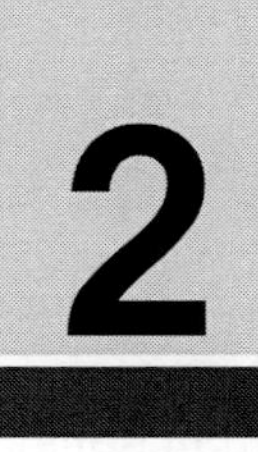

2 Faye Abdellah: Twenty-one Typology Nursing Problems

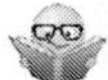 INTRODUCTION

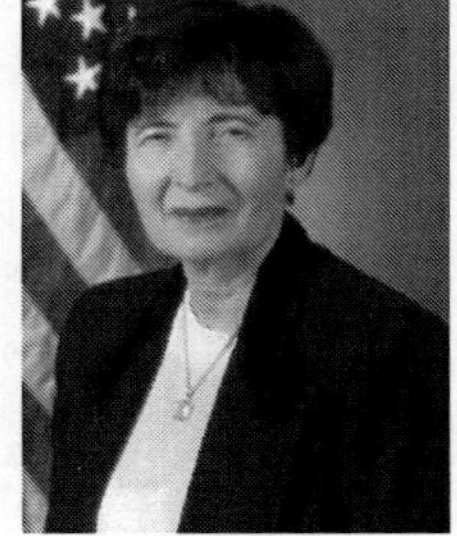
Faye Abdellah

She introduced the patient centered approach from the traditional disease focused nursing care. Furthermore, she also included the family member and elderly in the treatment plan.

Biography

- She was born on March 13, 1919, in New York City.
- She received Diploma in Nursing from Fitkin Memorial Hospital's School of Nursing in 1940 and Masters in Physiology in 1947.
- She worked as a public health nurse for around four decades with main focus on creating awareness among Americans regarding AIDS, violence and drug addiction.
- She is the first woman and nurse to serve as a Deputy Surgeon General for eight years before retiring in 1989.
- She received Doctorate in Education in 1955.
- She was honored as a 'living legend' by the American Academy of Nursing in 1994.

Major Concepts

A nursing problem which is faced by the client and family the nurse through her professional skills assist them to solve these problems. Abdellah identified 21 these nursing problems, hence her theory is also called ***21 Typology Nursing Problems.*** These problems are categorized into overt and covert problems. The overt problems are the one which is visible condition faced by patients and family, whereas the covert one is the hidden problems faced by them like emotional, interpersonal and sociocultural:

1. To maintain good hygiene and physical comfort
2. To promote optimal activity: Exercise, rest, sleep
3. To promote safety through prevention of accident, injury, or other trauma and through prevention of the spread of infection
4. To maintain good body mechanics and prevent and correct deformity

5. To facilitate the maintenance of a supply of oxygen to all body cells
6. To facilitate the maintenance of nutrition for all body cells
7. To facilitate the maintenance of elimination
8. To facilitate the maintenance of fluid and electrolyte balance
9. To recognize the physiologic responses of the body to disease conditions pathologic, physiologic, and compensatory
10. To facilitate the maintenance of regulatory mechanisms and functions
11. To facilitate the maintenance of sensory function
12. To identify and accept positive and negative expressions, feelings, and reactions
13. To identify and accept interrelatedness of emotions and organic illness
14. To facilitate the maintenance of effective verbal and nonverbal communication
15. To promote the development of productive interpersonal relationships
16. To facilitate progress toward achievement and personal spiritual goals
17. To create or maintain a therapeutic environment
18. To facilitate awareness of self as an individual with varying physical, emotional, and developmental needs
19. To accept the optimum possible goals in the light of limitations, physical and emotional
20. To use community resources as an aid in resolving problems that arise from illness
21. To understand the role of social problems as influencing factors in the cause of illness

These problems or needs are further divided into four levels: Basic to all patients, sustenal care needs, remedial care needs, and restorative care needs.

1. **Basic needs:** These are common to all individuals. The first four needs are falling in this category.
2. **Sustenal needs:** These mainly regulate the physiological and structural integrity of the body. The needs from fifth to 11 are coming under this category.
3. **Remedial needs:** This is related to the emotional and relationship of the clients with other and creation and maintenance of therapeutic environment. The needs from 12 to 18 come under this area.
4. **Restorative care needs:** This includes the relationship of sociocultural factors in the development of illness and proper use of community resources in order to solve the problems associated with diseases. The last three needs of the 21 typology of nursing problems come under this category.

The ten steps to identify the nursing problems are:

1. Learn to know the patient.
2. Sort out relevant and significant data.

3. Make generalizations about available data in relation to similar nursing problems presented by other patients.
4. Identify the therapeutic plan.
5. Test generalizations with the patient and make additional generalizations.
6. Validate the patient's conclusions about his nursing problems.
7. Continue to observe and evaluate the patient over a period of time to identify any attitudes and clues affecting his or her behavior.
8. Explore the patient and his or her family's reactions to the therapeutic plan and involve them in the plan.
9. Identify how the nurses feel about the patient's nursing problems.
10. Discuss and develop a comprehensive nursing care plan.

Metaparadigm in Nursing

Person: An individual who is the recipient of nursing care and has physical, emotional sociological needs.

Health: It is a state in which individuals have no needs to fulfill and the purpose of nursing is to achieve this state.

Environment: Though this is not clearly explained by Abdellah, she emphasized the importance of creating and maintenance of therapeutic environment.

Nursing: According to Abdellah, "Nursing is based on an art and science that moulds the attitudes, intellectual competencies, and technical skills of the individual nurse into the desire and ability to help people, sick or well, cope with their health needs."

Application of Faye Abdellah: 21 Typology Nursing Problems

Nursing education: Faye Abdellah's, 21 Typology Nursing Problems has been the framework for planning many nursing curriculum.

Nursing practice: Nurses use problem solving approaches to solve the identified nursing problems. It is primary designed for hospital setting, but can also apply in community areas.

Nursing research: She identified these 21 nursing problems after extensive research on various patients. Hence, this can act as a guide for various researches.

Nursing process according to Faye Abdellah: 21 Typology Nursing Problems

Phase	Nursing activities
Assessment	Data collection and identification of overt and covert problems of client and family
Nursing diagnosis	Grouping of one or more nursing problems to form broader nursing problems

Contd...

Contd...

Phase	Nursing activities
Planning	Determining nursing interventions as per the nursing problems
Implementation	Implementing the planned nursing actions
Evaluation	Checking the outcomes of nursing actions

Case Scenario: Mr X complaints about shortness of breath since last two weeks, decreased urine output and swelling over the body since last three months. The physician diagnosed him with chronic kidney disease.

Nursing assessment:

- Physical examination reveals pitting edema, respiratory rate 16 breaths per minute and urinary output around 800 ml per day.
- He is anxious and irritable about the disease and hospitalization.
- Having a past history of prostate resection.
- Less interested to interact with others.

Types of nursing problem	Nursing diagnosis	Nursing interventions
Basic to care	1. To maintain good hygiene and physical comfort	• Provide a semi-Fowlers position • Administer oxygen if required
Sustenal care needs	5. To facilitate the maintenance of a supply of oxygen to all body cells 8. To facilitate the maintenance of fluid and electrolyte balance	• Adequate rest • Positioning • Encourage for deep breathing and coughing exercises • Maintain intake and output record • Administer diuretics
Remedial needs	15. To promote the development of productive interpersonal relationships	• Positive reinforcement for the social interaction • Encouraged the health care and family members to have a calm and acceptable attitude towards patient
Restorative care needs	19. To accept the optimum possible goals in the light of limitations, physical and emotional	• Educate about the disease process and treatment plan • Encourage him to ventilate his feelings

Critique of the Theory

Clarity: All the theoretical statements are logical in nature. Much focus is given to the nursing and clients not VIE the client as a whole.

Simplicity: The concepts are very simple and easy to understand.

Generality: It can be easily reproduced in all the health care setting while working for the individuals, families and communities.

Empirical precision: The concepts in the theory can test in the research for the practicability and improve the various nursing interventions.

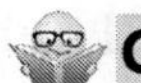

CONCLUSION

This theory is mainly focused on the clients need and nurses role in identification and solving these problems. Her theory has changed the entire nursing focus from disease to patient centered approach.

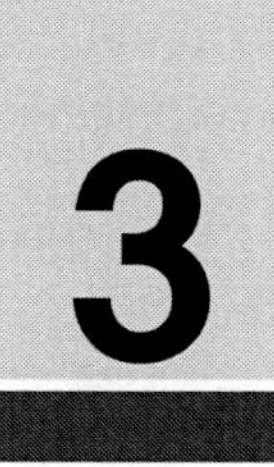

3 Lydia Eloise Hall: Core, Care and Cure Circles

'To look at and listen to self is often too difficult without the help of a significant figure (nurturer) who has learned how to hold up a mirror and sounding board to invite the behaver to look and listen to himself. If he accepts the invitation, he will explore the concerns in his acts and as he listens to his exploration through the reflection of the nurse, he may uncover in sequence his difficulties, the problem area, his problem, and eventually the threat which is dictating his out-of-control behavior.' –Lydia Eloise Hall (1965)

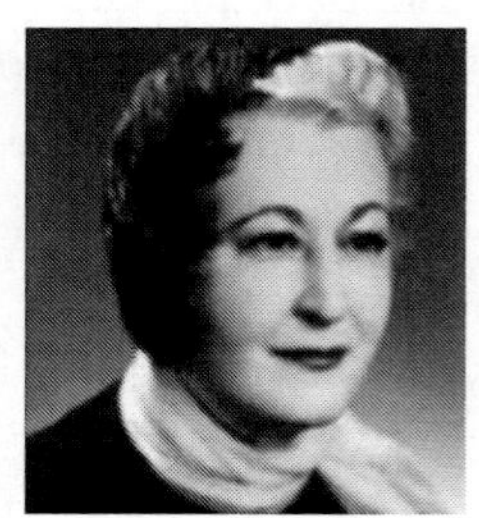

INTRODUCTION

Nursing theory in line with Lydia Hall is nothing short of revolutionary. In the 1960s, Hall put down her thoughts about nursing, in her own simple words. She did not consider herself as a nursing theorist, but instead she talked about her thoughts and remarkable ideas of nursing care as learned it over the years by her. These lead to the development of Hall's 'Care, Cure, Core Theory' also known as the 'Three Cs of Lydia Hall.' Nurses primarily function within these three realms: core, where nurses use theirselves to relate with the client; care, using hands on caring for the body and, cure, in the nurses' application of medical know-how.

Biography and Achievements

- Lydia Hall was born on September 21, 1906 in New York City and she grew up in Pennsylvania.
- She received her graduation from York Hospital School of Nursing in Pennsylvania in 1927.
- She earned her Bachelor of Science and Master of Arts from Teachers College, Columbia University in 1937 and 1942, respectively.
- She died on February 27, 1969 of heart disease in Queens Hospital of New York.
- She worked with the Visiting Nurse Service of New York from 1941 to 1947.
- She worked as a faculty in Fordham Hospital School of Nursing from 1947 to 1950.

- Also worked as a faculty at Teachers College.
- She also involved in US Health Service research activities.
- Hall provided volunteer service to New York Board of Education, Youth Aid, and other community associations.
- She received the Teachers College Nursing Alumni Award in 1967.
- She established the Loeb Center for Nursing and Rehabilitation at Montefiore Hospital in Bronx, New York.
- She provided direct care to clients and coordinated needed services.
- Practice model was validated over a 5-year-time with a reduction in hospital readmission.
- Hall career interests revolved around public health nursing, pediatric cardiology cardiovascular nursing, and nursing of long-term illnesses.
- Hall authored 21 publications and many articles and her nursing theory were published in the early to middle 1960s.

METAPARADIGM OF THE THEORY

- **Individual/Person:**
  - The main focus of nursing care in Lydia E Hall's work is the human being who is 16 years older and past the acute stage of long-term illness.
  - She emphasizes the importance of an individual/person as unique, capable of growth and learning, and requiring a total person approach.
  - Client is composed of body, pathology, and person.
  - Individuals set their own goals and they are capable of learning and growing and achieve their maximum potential.
- **Health:**
  - It can be inferred to be a state of self-awareness with conscious selection of behaviors that are optimal for that person.
  - She stresses the need to help the individual explore the meaning of his behavior to identify and overcome problems through developing self-identity and maturity.
  - She considered becoming ill is the behavior.
- **Nursing:**
  - Nursing is identified as consisting participation in the care, core, and cure aspects of client care.
  - Care is the sole function of nurses and core and cure are shared with other members of the health care team. Major purpose of nursing care is to achieve an interpersonal relationship with the person which facilitate the development of core.
- **Environment/society:**
  - The concept of environment is dealt within relation to the individual/ person.

- Hall developed the concept of Loeb Center because she assumed that the hospital environment during treatment of acute illness creates a difficult psychological experience for the ill person.
- Loeb Center focuses on providing an environment that is conducive to self-development. In such a setting, action of the nurses is for assisting the individual in achieving a personal goal.

Assumptions

- The client holds the motivation and energy necessary for healing.
- The three aspects of nursing should be viewed as interrelated but not viewed as functioning independently.
- The three aspects interact and the circles change size, based on the patient's progress.

Concepts of the Theory

- *Behavior:* According to Hall behavior as everything that is said or done. Behavior is dictated by conscious and unconscious feelings.
- *Reflection:* She defines reflection as a Rogerian method of communication in which selected verbalizations of client is repeated back to him with different phraseology, to invite him to explore feelings further.
- *Self-awareness:* She defines self-awareness is the state of being that nurses try to help their client's achieve. The more self-awareness individuals have of their feelings, the more control they have over their behavior.
- *Phases of medical care:* She divides medical care into 2 phases; biologically critical and evaluate the follow-up. During the first phase, the client receives intensive medical care and multiple diagnostic. It lasts a few days to a week or more and is the period when physicians plan treatment that help the patient reach the second phase. The second phase begins when doctor starts giving only follow-up care. She defines second stage of illness as the non-acute recovery phase of illness. This stage is helpful for learning and rehabilitation. The need for medical care is minimal but nurturing and learning is great. So this is the ideal time for wholly professional nursing.
- *Wholly professional nursing:* Wholly professional nursing means nursing care given exclusively by professional registered nurses educated in the behavioral sciences who take responsibility and opportunity to coordinate and deliver the total care of clients like nurturing, teaching and advocacy in the promotion of healing.

THEORY ASSERTION

Lydia Hall's model has three components which are represented by three independent but interconnected circles. These three circles are—the core, the care, and the cure. The size of each circle constantly varies and depends on the state of the client. The size of the circles represents the degree to which the client is progressing in each of the three areas. The professional nurse at this time is able to help the client reach the core of his problem through the closeness provided by the care aspect of nursing. She developed this model in 1960s.

Care Circle

- The care circle represents the nurturing component of nursing.
- Exclusive function of nurses is the care and nurses nurture clients.
- Nurturing involves using the factors that make up the concept of mothering (care and comfort of the individual) and provide for teaching-learning activities.
- The nurse-patient relationship is therapeutic in itself.
- Professional nursing care is the most important need of chronically ill patients.
- The professional nurse provides bodily care for the client and helps the client to complete such basic daily biological functions as eating, elimination, bathing, and dressing. When providing this care, the nurse's goal is to provide comfort to client.
- Nurses help clients meet their needs when assistance is required to them.
- Teaching is a part of caring.
- Nurses form interpersonal relationships with clients.
- A hand on care creates an atmosphere of trust and open communication between clients and nurses.
- It is based on natural and biological science.

Cure Circle

- It is based on the pathological and therapeutic sciences.
- The cure process is shared with medicine.
- Nurses apply their knowledge of disease to assist with the medical plan of care and educate the clients and their families about the process of illness.
- By performing medical tasks nurses assist doctors.
- Nurses help clients and families adhere to and understand the treatment ordered by doctors.
- Nurses act as client advocates.

Core Circle

- It is based on the social science.
- The core is shared with other members of the health team like psychologists, social workers, clergy and the community.
- The professional nurse, by developing an interpersonal relationship with the client (mainly through effective communication), is able to help the client verbally express feelings regarding the disease process and its

effects. Through such expression, the client is able to gain self-identity and further develop maturity.

- Nurses help clients understand their roles in the rehabilitation process.
- By the use of **reflective technique** (acting as a mirror to the client) the professional nurse, helps the client look at and explore feelings regarding his current health status and related potential changes in lifestyle.
- **Motivations** are discovered through the process of bringing into awareness the feelings being experienced. With this awareness, the client is now able to make conscious decisions based on understood and accepted feelings and motivation.

Lydia Hall's Care, Cure, Core model was the first to stress that the whole individual needed care and only professional nurses should give care to clients. It included not only care of clients but also integrated care of their families and advocated for community involvement. The nurse is present in all the circles of the model of Lydia Hall. The main focus of the nurse's role is on the care circle. This is where the nurse acts as a professional in order to help the client meet his needs and to attain a sense of balance.

Cure circle is dominant during the acute phase of disease, but core and care circle is dominant in the sub-acute phase of disease. The care circle also will be dominant during rehabilitation and follow-up phases and immediate post-acute care.

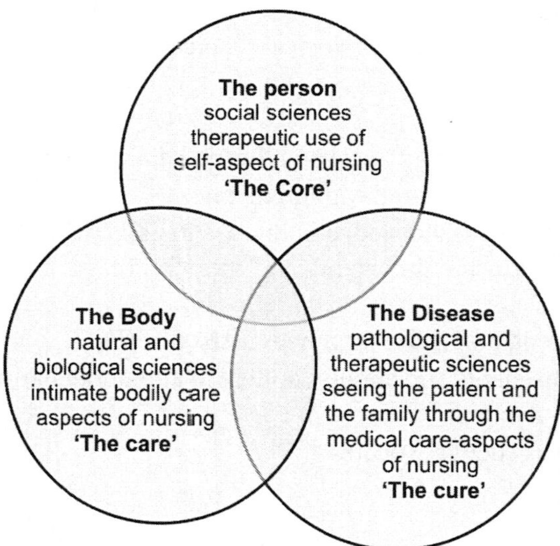

Fig. 3.1: Core, care and cure model

Thus, nursing could be most effective when the client was out of biological crisis and needed help with care and core issues. Since the nurse physically takes care of the body (care) of the client by touching or 'the laying on of hands' she develops a nurturing/fostering relationship with the client and is in the perfect position to teach the client about his own feelings (core). The nurse reflects the client's feelings back to him in hope that this will lead to self-awareness in the client. It is through this self-awareness of the client that Hall says, 'Healing might be hastened'. Hall admits that there is no conclusive evidence that this self-awareness hastens healing, but she does point out the positive outcomes that are associated with the Loeb Center.

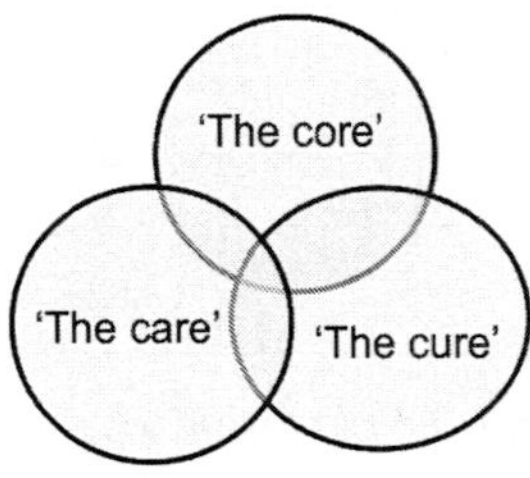

Fig. 3.2: Acute patient care

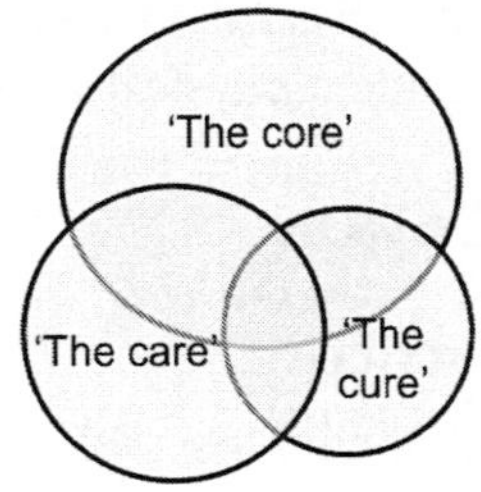

'The core'
'The care'
'The cure'

Fig. 3.3: Sub-acute phase of disease

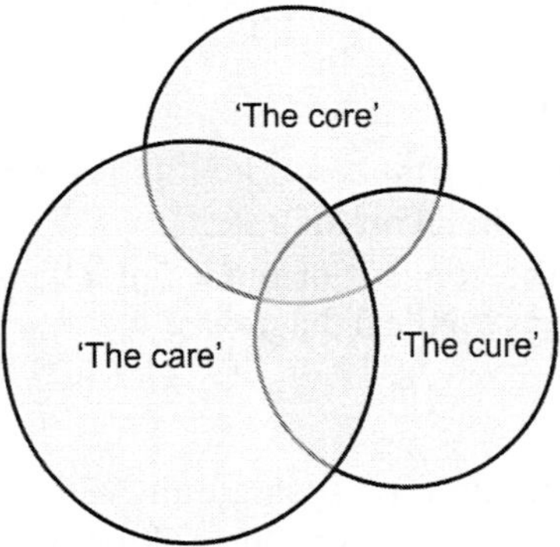

Fig. 3.4: Immediate postacute care

Hall's Theory and Nursing Process

- *Assessment phase:* It involves collection of data about the health status of the person. According to Hall, the process of data collection is benefit for the client rather than for the benefit of the nurse.
- *Nursing diagnosis phase:* It is the statement of the client's need or problem area.
- *Outcomes and planning:* It involves setting priorities and mutually establishing client-centered outcomes and goals and the client decides the highest priority and also what outcomes and goals are desirable for him for the recovery.
- *Implementation phase:* It involves the actual establishment of the plan of care.
- *Evaluation phase:* It is the process of asserting the clients progress toward the health goals. It is directed toward deciding whether or not the client is successful in reaching the established goals. Evaluation is done on the basis of the following questions:

- Is the patient learning 'who he is, where he wants to go and how he wants to go there?
- Is the patient learning to understand and explore the feelings that underlie behavior?
- Is the nurse helping the patient see motivations more clearly?
- Are the patient's goals congruent with the medical regime? Is the patient successful in meeting the goals?
- Is the patient physically more comfortable?

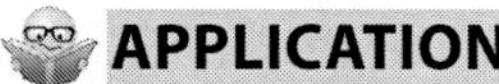

APPLICATION

Nursing Practice

- Lydia Hall's theory resembles the nursing model of primary care.
- Hall's concepts of nurses being relevant and applicable ideas and are accountable and responsible for their own practice. Concerns for these concepts demonstrate support for Hall's theory.

Nursing Education

- Hall's theory gives importance to definite ideas regarding nursing care provided by a professional nursing staff.
- Hall emphasized the concept of nurses practicing as practical doctors 'Nursing diagnosis vs Medical diagnosis'.

Nursing Research

Hall's theory implementation in nursing units within the United States was not found outside the Loeb Center. Given the changes in health care and current Medicare and Medicaid policies and procedures, it may be difficult to further test Hall's original assertion that wholly professional nursing care will hasten recovery.

Limitations

- In this theory acute stage illness clients are not included
- Only refers clients above 16 years
- Reflection is only tool of therapeutic communication
- Only in cure circle family is mentioned
- Her theory relates only to those who are ill
- This theory was not satisfied with concept of 'team nursing'.

Critique of the Theory

- *Simplicity:* This theory is simple and easily understood. The major concepts and relationships are limited and clear. The theory is easily understood and is indigenous to nursing as the language used to define and describe the theory is simple.

- *Generality:* The most serious fault of Hall's theory of nursing it is limited generality. Hall devotes her theory to adult individuals who are ill.
- *Empirical Precision:* Hall's theory has been tested at two other facilities and has been found successful. These two facilities only care for adults, mainly those over 65 years of age. Therefore, empirical precision of Hall's theory continues to be limited, further testing in facilities not caring for adults will still be needed.
- *Derivable Consequences:* The theory provides a general framework for nursing and the concepts are within the domain of nursing, although the aspects of Cure and Core are shared with other professionals and family members. Application of the theory in practice has produced valued outcomes in all three areas.

CLINICAL APPLICATION OF HALL'S CORE, CARE AND CURE CIRCLES

Assessment

Minnu is a 25-year-old post-graduating cricket player in a university. Unfortunately, while on her way to her match, she was involved in an automobile accident in which her left arm was crushed and his left leg was injured. There was concern about possible internal injuries but luckily there was none. The required surgeries have been completed for her left arm and foot; she is now in physical therapy to deal with the effects of the accident and her recent immobility.

Care	Core	Cure
• Physically, the remarkable findings are her left arm is in an orthopedic device to stabilize it and encourage bone healing. • She is left handed but has learned to compensate with her right hand for most activities of daily living. She needs minor assistance for dressing. • She is rapidly gaining confidence in her ability to provide for her own physical care.	She is looking at the floor, tells you, her nurse that she is going home tomorrow? And share your observation that she is not looking very happy about the prospect. Minnu says' yes, I am doing okay here but I am scared about going back to school. How will take notes and tests? It Looks like I have totally messed up cricket team. I am more worried with grades. I have to do well in school, or else I will not be able to graduate this year. I am scared that I cannot fully use my dominant arm; I am also very worried with physical therapy.	The surgical incision on her left arm and left leg has healed and she is beginning to bear weight on the foot. There are no problems with her hydration or elimination, skin is intact with good skin turgor, all the vital signs and laboratory values are within normal levels. She is finishing her antibiotics.

Nursing Diagnosis: Reluctant to be discharged associated with concerns about abilities to successfully meet academic expectations (Core Circle).

Outcome: Postgraduate in College and meet academic expectations.

Goals: Regain uring left arm as much as possible (Care and cure circles). And successful completion of academic expectation/performance to be able to postgraduate in college (Core Circle).

Implementation: The school nurse is most likely to involved at this point. Arrange physical therapy sessions for her around school schedule. Take notes with right hand. Arrange to have extra time for her for written tests. Provide listening ear to help, Minnu is dealing with frustrations that are bound to arise.

Evaluation by Using Hall's Five Questions

- Yes, she wants to postgraduate this year and now is not likely for her to play again for the cricket team, so she has changed her focus to academics (Core).
- She verbalized her feelings and concerns on what happened to her, and at the possibility that she may not regain full use of her dominant arm. She has also recognized that her initial resistance to physical therapy was based on fear (Core).
- The nurse at the hospital helped her to verbalize her concerns about being discharged. The school nurse helps her decide to ask for extra time for tests since she writes slower with her right hand. She will do anything to graduate.
- Her goals are congruent with the medical regimen and she is meeting those goals. Physical therapy has been arranged for her after school, she has learned to use a laptop computer with one hand to take notes, do homework and take tests, her teachers have been accommodating about testing time, some have been willing to give oral tests for her (Cure and Core).
- Physically, her arm continues to be uncomfortable and her foot aches at times. As a total individual, she is comfortable that she is successfully refocusing her efforts to meet her objective of post-graduating in college (Care and Core).

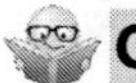

CONCLUSION

Hall used her knowledge of psychiatry and nursing experiences in the Loeb Center as a framework for formulating the Care, Core and Cure Theory. This theory gives importance on the importance of the total client rather than looking at one part or aspect. There is also emphasis give on all three aspects of the theory, the three Cs, functioning together.

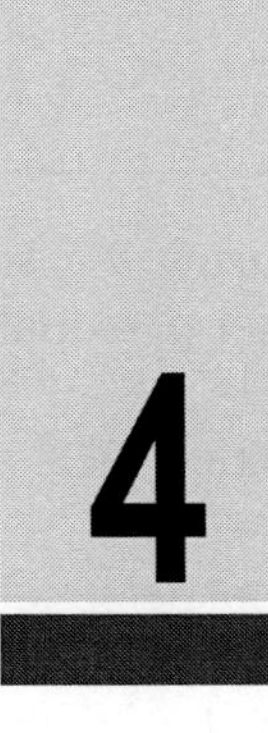

4 Virginia Henderson: Fourteen Components of Basic Nursing Care

'The nurse is temporarily the consciousness of the unconscious, the love of life for the suicidal, the leg of the amputee, the eyes of the newly blind, a means of locomotion for the infant, knowledge and confidence for the mother, the mouthpiece for those too weak or withdrawn to speak and so on.'

–Virginia Henderson

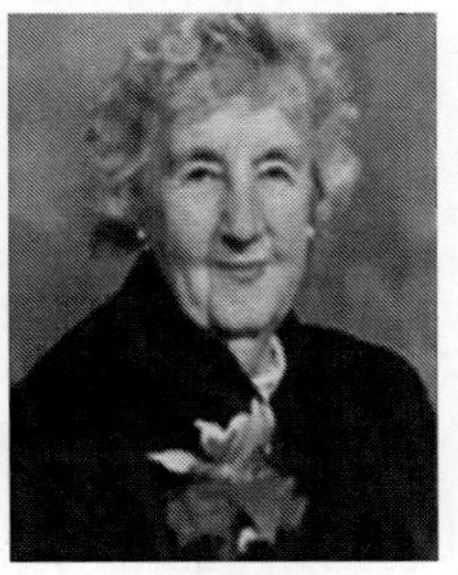

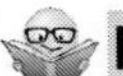 INTRODUCTION

The Nursing Need Theory was developed by Virginia Avenel Henderson who is known as *'First Lady of Nursing,' 'First Truly International Nurse,' 'The Nightingale of Modern Nursing'* and *'Modern-Day Mother of Nursing.'* Her goal was to define the unique focus of nursing practice and not to develop a nursing theory. This theory mainly focuses on the importance of increasing the patient's independence to hasten their progress in the hospital. Henderson's theory given emphasizes on the basic human needs and how nurses can assist the clients in meeting those needs.

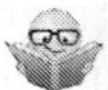 BIOGRAPHY AND ACHIEVEMENTS

- Virginia Avenel Henderson was born on November 30, 1897 in Kansas City, Missouri, the 5th of eight children of Daniel Brosius Henderson and Lucy Minor Abbot.
- She did her early schooling from Virginia.
- She developed interest in nursing in 1918 because of World War I.
- She was graduated from Army School of Nursing, in Washington, DC in 1921 and then worked as a staff nurse of the Henry Street Visiting Nurse Service in New York City.
- She began teaching in Norfolk Protestant Hospital, Virginia in 1922.
- She served as teaching supervisor in the clinics of Strong Memorial Hospital, Ronchester, New York in 1929.
- She received her BS and MA degrees in nursing education from Teacher's College at Columbia University in 1932 and 1934 respectively and then taught from 1934 until 1948.

- Henderson revised Bertha Harmer's classic textbook of nursing for its 4th edition and later wrote the 5th edition which contains her personal definition of nursing.
- She joined at Yale School of Nursing as Research Associates since 1953.
- She was recipient of multiple Honorary Doctoral degrees.
- She included physiological and psychological principles into her personal concept of nursing .
- She also concluded that 'A definition of nursing should imply an appreciation' of the principles of physiological balance. From Bernard's theory, she also gained an appreciation for psychosomatic medicine and its implications for nursing.
- In Henderson's 14 components of nursing care a co-relation with Abraham Maslow's Hierarchy of Needs is seen. The components which begin with physical needs and progress to the psychological components
- She died in 1996 at the Connecticut Hospice, aged 98.

EVOLUTION OF THEORY

- Virginia A. Henderson was the theorist who dedicated her career to defining nursing practice.
- She believed that an occupation that affects human life must outline its functions particularly if it is said to be a profession.
- Her ideas about definition of nursing were influenced by nursing education and practice by her students and colleagues at Columbia University School of Nursing, and by distinguished nursing leaders on that time.
- Two events are the basis for her development of definition of nursing :
  - First, she participated in the revision of a nursing text book, *'Textbooks of the Principles and Practice of Nursing'* written with Bertha Harmer in 1922 that time Henderson realized the need to be clear about the functions of the nurse.
  - Second, she knew that the many states had no provision for nursing licensure to ensure safe and competent care for the consumers.
- Henderson disagreed with the definition of nursing practice given by American Nurses Association (ANA) in 1932 and 1937 publication.
- Henderson research work allows for the modification of the ANA definition in 1955.

ASSUMPTIONS

- Nurse provides care to patients until patients can care for themselves once again.
- Patients desire to return to health or a peaceful death and they will act in such a way to achieve this.
- Individuals will perform activities which leading to health if they have the knowledge, capacity or will.

- The individual's goal and the nurse's goal are similar.
- The 14 basic needs symbolize nursing's basic function.
- Nurses are willing to serve and that 'nurses will devote themselves to the patient day and night.'
- Nurse is an independent practitioner.
- Nurses should be educated at the university level in both arts and sciences.
- She also believes that mind and body are inseparable. It is implied that the mind and body are interrelated.

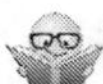 MAJOR CONCEPTS AND DEFINITIONS

The major concepts of Virginia Henderson's needs theory relate to the metaparadigm.

Mataparadigm of Henderson's Need Theory

- **Individual:**
  - Persons have basic needs (14 components) that are component of health.
  - Individual require assistance to achieve health or recovery or a peaceful death.
  - According to her mind and body are inseparable and interrelated.
  - She considers the biological, psychological, sociological, and spiritual components. The theory presents the patient as a sum of parts with biopsychosocial needs.
- **Environment:**
  - Environment is a setting in which an individual learns unique pattern for living.
  - All external conditions (light, temperature, air movement, atmospheric pressure, proper waste disposal, absence of injurious chemicals, cleanliness of surroundings) influences and that affect life and its development.
  - She believes that environment are that individuals in relation to families but minimally discusses the impact of the community on the individual and family.
  - Basic nursing care involves providing conditions under which the patient can perform the 14 activities unaided.
- **Health:**
  - Individual's ability to function independently 14 basic needs.
  - Nurses need to stress promotion of health and prevention and cure of disease.
  - Good health is a challenge which is affected by age, cultural background, physical, and intellectual capacities, and emotional balance.

- **Nursing:**
  - Nurses temporarily assist an individual who is sick or well and not able to fulfill their basic needs.
  - Nurses assists and supports the individual in life activities to help to attain independence.
  - The nurse is supposed to carry out physician's therapeutic plan.
  - The nurse's creativity in planning for care result in individualized care.
  - 'Nurse should have knowledge to practice individualized care and should be a scientific problem solver.'
  - Nurse functions in relation with the patient, physician and the health team:
    - *Nurse-Patient Relationship:* As a substitute for the patient, as a helper for the patient, and as a partner with the patient
    - *Nurse-Physician Relationship*
    - *Nurse as a Member of the Health Team*
  - Her definition of nursing is:

'The unique function of the nurse is to assist the individual, sick or well, in the performance of those activities contributing to health or its recovery (or to peaceful death) that he would perform unaided if he had the necessary strength, will or knowledge. And to do this in such a way as to help him gain independence as rapidly as possible.'

–Henderson, 1966

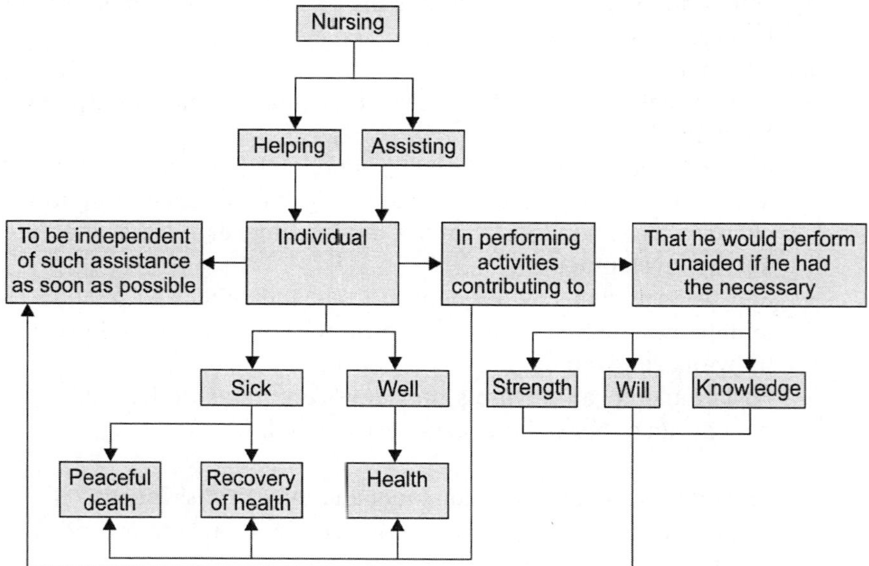

Fig. 4.1: Virginia Henderson's concept of nursing

Fourteen Basic Human Needs

Henderson's 14 components of basic nursing care as follows:

1. Breathe normally.
2. Eat and drink adequately.
3. Eliminate body wastes.
4. Move and maintain desirable positions.
5. Sleep and rest.
6. Select suitable clothing—dress and undress.
7. Maintain body temperature within normal range by adjusting clothing and modifying the environment.
8. Keep the body clean and well-groomed and protect the integument.
9. Avoid dangers in the environment and avoid injuring others.
10. Communicate with others in expressing emotions, needs, fears, or opinions.
11. Worship according to one's faith.
12. Work in such a way that there is a sense of accomplishment.
13. Play or participate in various forms of recreation.
14. Learn, discover, or satisfy the curiosity that leads to normal development and health and use the available health facilities.

The first nine components are physiological. The tenth and fourteenth are psychological aspects of communicating and learning. The eleventh component is spiritual and moral. The twelfth and thirteenth components are sociologically oriented to occupation and recreation.

 COMPARISON WITH MASLOW'S HIERARCHY OF NEED

The 14 basic need can be applied or compared to Abraham Maslow's Hierarchy of Needs.

Maslow's	Henderson's
Physiological needs	1. Breathe normally 2. Eat and drink adequately 3. Eliminate body waste 4. Move and maintain desirable posture 5. Sleep and rest 6. Select suitable clothing 7. Maintain body temperature 8. Keep body clean and well-groomed and protect the skin
Safety needs	9. Avoid environmental dangers and avoid injuring other
Belongingness and love needs	10. Communicate with others 11. Worship according to one's faith
Esteem needs	12. Work at something providing a sense of accomplishment 13. Play or participate in various forms of recreation 14. Learn, discover, or satisfy curiosity

 CHARACTERISTIC OF HENDERSON'S THEORY

- This theory can interrelate concepts in such a way as to create a different.
- Concepts of fundamental human needs, biophysiology, culture, and interaction, communication and is borrowed from other discipline (Maslow's Hierarchy of human needs); concept of interaction-communication (nurse-patient relationship).
- Theories must be logical in nature.
- Henderson's definition and components are logical and the 14 components are a guide for in reaching the chosen goal by the individual and nurse.
- This theory is relatively simple yet generalizable with some limitation.
- Henderson's work can be applied to the health of individuals of all age group.
- Theories can be the bases for hypotheses that can be tested. Her definition of nursing cannot be viewed as theory; therefore, it is impossible to generate testable hypotheses. However some questions to investigate the definition of nursing and the 14 components may be useful.
- Theories contribute to and assist in increasing the general body of knowledge within the discipline through the research implemented to validate them.
- Henderson's ideas of nursing practice are well-accepted throughout the world as a basis for nursing care. However, the impact of the definition and components has not been established through research.
- Theories can be utilized by practitioners to guide and improve their practice. Ideally the nurse would improve nursing practice by using her definition and 14 components to improve the health of individuals and thus reduce illness.
- Theories must be consistent with other validated theories, laws, and principles but will leave open unanswered questions that need to be investigated.

 HENDERSON'S THEORY AND NURSING PROCESS

Virginia Avenel Henderson views the nursing process as 'really the application of the logical approach to the solution of a problem. The steps are those of the scientific method.' 'Nursing process stresses the science of nursing rather than the mixture of science and art on which it seems effective health care service of any kind is based.'

Nursing process	Henderson's 14 components and definiton of nursing
Nursing assessment	1. Assess needs of human being based in the Henderson's 14 components of basic nursing care
Nursing diagnosis	2. Analysis: Compare data to knowledge base of health and disease

Contd...

Contd...

Nursing process	Henderson's 14 components and definiton of nursing
Nursing plan	3. Nurse identify individual's ability to meet his/her own needs with or without assistance, taking into consideration strength, will or knowledge 4. Prioritization of needs is done by the nurse together with the client 5. Long-term goal: Optimal independence 6. Short-term goals: Successful activities as directed to the fulfillment of the long-term goals
Nursing implementation	7. Document how the nurse can assist the individual, sick or well 8. Assist the sick or well person in to performance of activities in meeting human needs to maintain health, recover from illness, or to aid in peaceful death
Nursing process	9. Implementation based on the physiological principles, age, cultural background, emotional balance, and physical and intellectual capacities 10. Nurse carry out treatment prescribed by the physician
Nursing evaluation	11. Henderson's 14 components and definition of nursing 12. Use the acceptable definition of nursing and appropriate laws related to the practice of nursing 13. The quality of care is affected by the preparation and ability of the nurse rather that the amount of hours of care 14. Successful outcomes of nursing care are based on the speed with which or degree to which the client performs independently the activities of daily living

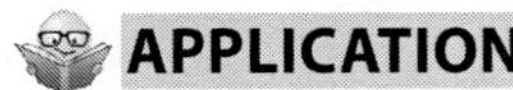

Nursing Practice

- With the birth of Henderson's theory, it guided the nurses to remain faithful to his/her functional roles and professional boundaries.
- Henderson's theory helps the nurses to assist the patient move to an independent state by assessing, planning, implementing and evaluating each of 14 components of basic nursing care.
- It also helps the nurses to assist the client to perform activities to maintain heath, to recover from illness or to aid in peaceful death.
- The practice of regulating nursing practice through licensure is evident today because of Henderson's effort. For example, in the Philippines, the Board of Nursing which is the 'ultimate authority in regulating the nursing profession in the country' through the Professional Regulation Commission, has expressed its mission to 'lead nursing development to its highest level of excellence for the health and safety of the public.'
- The concept of nursing by Henderson is universal. It was adopted by WHO Expert Committee on Nursing Practice in 1995.

Nursing Education

- The book *Principles and Practice of Nursing* describes definition to nursing and this book been used as a basic text in many schools of nursing.
- Henderson's theory is given in curriculum for nursing.
- Henderson's curriculum helps in structured learning experiences which are goal directive.
- This theory helps the nurses in creative thinking.
- In the Philippine setting, the basic nursing curriculum is based on Henderson ideas and is evident in the four year nursing programs today.
- Henderson (1977) gave emphasis on interdisciplinary education and fostering a humanistic concept of health care.

Nursing Research

- Henderson's theory gives a source for educational research.
- Henderson's basic needs serve as a source for the nursing research.
- This theory helps to formulate the questions in nursing research.
- Nicely, Bruce, DeLario and Ginger (2011) written an article. In this article the theory of Virginia Henderson was utilized creatively in the practice and principles of nursing as applied to organ donation after brain death in the clinical practice. This shows how the theory can be feasible in clinical research.
- Evelyn Adam who is a Canadian nurse, extended the work of Henderson, by developing concepts integrated into a conceptual model (George, 1995).

LIMITATION

- There is no theoretical association between physiological and other characteristics of human.
- No awareness of holistic nature of human being.
- Her 14 components are prioritized; the connections among the components are not well-defined.
- Dying process is not well explained in her theory and the role of the nurse.
- This theory lacks interrelation of factors and the influence of nursing care.

CRITIQUE

- **Simplicity:** This theory is complex rather than simplistic. It contains many variables and several descriptive and explanatory relationships. Not associated with structural organizations within a framework or model form to enhance simplicity.
- **Clarity:** Definitions and concepts are clear and self-explanatory.
- **Generality:** Henderson's theory is generable because it is broad in scope. It attempts to include the function of all nurses and all patients in their various interrelationships and interdependence.

- **Empirical precision:** Theory is used in many research studies has been found testable and applicable in research. This theory provides a theory based on reality.
- **Derivable consequences:** Henderson's perspective has been useful in promoting new ideas and in furthering conceptual development of emerging theorist. She has discussed the importance of nag's interdependence from and interdependence with, other branches of health care field. This theory is helpful in curriculum development and made great contribution in promoting the importance of research in the clinical practice of nursing.

CLINICAL APPLICATION OF VIRGINIA HENDERSON'S NEED THEORY

Master Ruhan, an 8-year-old admitted to orthopedic ward with fractures due to fall down form height while playing. He was placed on cast in right leg which limited his movement and stitches in wounds in left hand and jaw.

Assessment

By using 14 basic needs Henderson the nurse would able to understand his condition.

Planning

By using Henderson's concept the nurse would able to prioritize her intervention towards the attainment of independence through the performance of the basic human needs.

Implementation

On top of the nurse performing as a substitute for the patient, actions must also be directed in having participated gradually over his care.

Evaluation

Upon entertaining this phase, the entire process is evaluated and new goals are to be formulated.

Fourteen Basic Needs of Master Ruhan

1. **Breathing normally:** Respiratory assessment would need to be done to ensure proper breathing and absence of pneumonia or other respiratory illness in Ruhan. Normal breathing is just the first step to ensuring the well-being of him.
2. **Eating and drinking adequately:** The nurse should assure that Ruhan is receiving adequate intake food and fluid. The nurse should monitor intake/output chart also.

3. **Eliminate body waste:** As he is non-ambulatory and confined to bed it is very important to ensure the elimination pattern every day and bowl sound.
4. **Move and maintain desirable positions:** The nurse should ensure that he is not lying in the same position for long periods of time. In order to prevent skin breakdown frequent position changes (every 2 hour) are necessary.
5. **Sleep and rest:** Adequate sleep and rest are essential for him. The nurse should instruct to her mother about sleep routines. It may be necessary for the mother to ask help from family members for assistance.
6. **Select suitable clothes—dress and undress:** The nurse should ensure that he has season appropriate clothing. Change his dressing as it become wet.
7. **Maintain body temperature within normal range by adjusting clothing and modifying environment:** The nurse should provide information to the mother regarding importance of maintain temperature in the room. The nurse opens the windows and provides the mother with a fan for better air movement.
8. **Keep the body clean and well-groomed and protect the integument:** The nurse should assist the mother in bathing him and applying lotion to the back to prevent skin breakdown. The mother should also be taught the importance of cleanliness and the consequences of not protecting the skin.
9. **Avoid dangers in the environment and avoid injuring others:** The nurse should educate the mother on the dangers of heat exhaustion and the importance of a clean, cool environment. Emphasis should be placed on cleanliness of the room and the environment.
10. **Communicate with others in expressing emotions, needs, fears, or opinions:** The nurse should provide therapeutic communication for the mother and Ruhan. Regularly scheduled visits to the doctor and pediatrician should also be encouraged.
11. **Worship according to one's faith**: Importance of faith should be conveyed to the mother. He can always turn to their God for strength and wisdom.
12. **Work in such a way that there is a sense of accomplishment**: The mother should be taught to feel a sense of accomplishment after completing everyday tasks. These accomplishments will boost self-esteem and provide inner peace.
13. **Play or participate in various forms of recreation**: Recreation is very important for his growth and development. The nurse should encourage the mother to take him in the park when he is physically ready. Laughter is good medicine. The mother should be encouraged to interact with him in fun, playful ways.

14. **Learn, discover or satisfy the curiosity that leads to normal development and health and use the available health facilities**: The nurse should provide the mother with a list of health facilities that would be of assistance to him.

 CONCLUSION

She concluded that, 'No profession, occupation or industry in this age can evaluate adequately or improve its practice without research.' Henderson's considers that research in nursing is essential for nursing practice in the age of technological advancements. The 'concept of nursing' as Henderson described it has multidimensional facets. Henderson's definition of Nursing is not only applicable in nursing practice but is also important in the nursing academic and realm of nursing research.

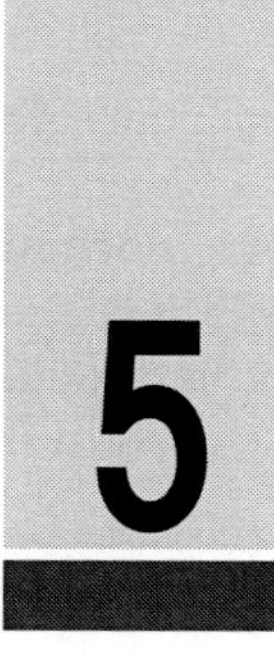

5 Dorothy E Johnson: Behavioral System Model

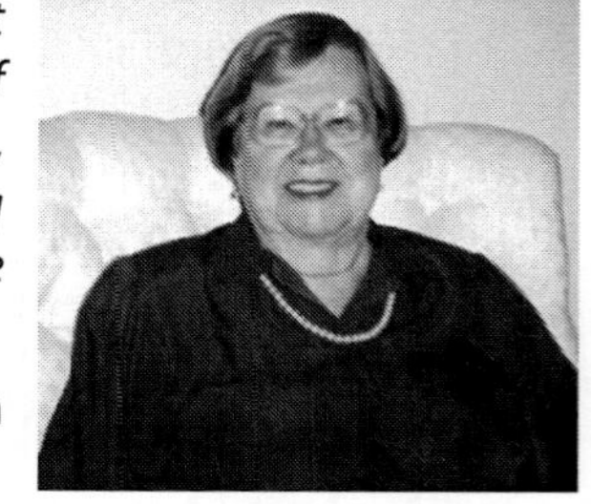

'All of us, scientists and practicing processionals, must turn our attention to practice and ask questions of that practice. We must be inquisitive and inquiring, seeking the fullest and truest possible understanding of the theoretical and practical problems we encounter'.

–Dorothy E Johnson

INTRODUCTION

Dorothy Johnson is well-known for her 'Behavioral System Model,' which was first proposed in 1968. It describes the development of efficient and effective behavioral functioning in the client to prevent illness and she stresses the importance of research-based knowledge about the effect of nursing care on clients. Johnson's behavioral system model is a conceptual model that views the person as a behavioral system. The behavioral system is made up of all patterned, repetitive, and purposeful ways of behavior that characterize each one's life. Her theory defined Nursing as 'an external regulatory force which acts to preserve the organization and integration of the patients' behaviors at an optimum level under those conditions in which the behavior constitutes a threat to the physical or social health, or in which illness is found.' The behavioral system encompasses seven subsystems that carry out specialized tasks or functions needed to maintain the integrity of the whole behavioral system and manage its relationship to the environment.

Biography and Achievements

- Dorothy E Johnson was born on August 21, 1919 in Savannah, Georgia, youngest of 7 children.
- She completed her Associates Degree in 1938 from Armstrong Junior College in Savannah, Georgia.
- She received her BSN from Vanderbilt University in Nashville, Tennessee in 1942.
- She received her Masters in public health (MPH) from Harvard University, Boston, Massachusetts in 1948.
- After graduation, she worked in public health nursing for one year (1943–1944) and began to teach (assistant professor in Pediatric Nursing) at Vanderbilt University in their school of nursing.

- After 5 years, from 1949 she moved to California where she was an instructor for pediatrics in the school of nursing at the University of California, Los Angeles (UCLA). She worked at UCLA until she retired in 1978, except for one year in 1955 when Dorothy took sabbatical from UCLA to teach in Vellore, South India at the Christian Medical College School of Nursing.
- She was Chairperson on the California's Nurses Association (1965-1967) that developed a position statement for specifications for clinical specialists.
- Her publications include four books, more than 30 articles, and many other papers, reports, proceedings and monographs.
- She received many honors.
- She died in February 1999 at the age of 80.

Theoretical Background

- She was influenced mainly by Florence Nightingale's book and notes on Nursing.
- Johnson used the work of behavioral scientist, psychology, sociology, and ethnology to form her seven subsystems.
- She also relied on the system theory and used concepts and definitions from Rapport, Chin, Von Bertalanffy, and Buckley.

Behavior System Model

- In this model she conceptualizes an individual as a behavioral system, in which the behavior of the individual as a whole is the focus.
- The patient is defined as a behavioral system is divided into seven subsystems that are open, linked, and interrelated. Balance is maintained within a person's subsystems. These seven subsystems are continuously changing through maturation, experience, and learning.
- Each subsystem is comprised of four structural characteristics.
- An imbalance in each results in disequilibrium.
- The nurses' goal is to help the client to obtain and maintain equilibrium, in which the individual is in harmony with themselves and the environment.

Metaparadigm of the Theory

- *Nursing:* Nursing is as an external regulatory force—the goal is to maintain and restore an individual's behavioral systems balance through imposing temporary regulatory or control mechanisms through resources, i.e. a primary goal of nursing that is to foster equilibrium within the individual. Nursing activities do not depend on medical authority but are complementary to medicine.
- *Person/Human being:* Johnson considers human beings having two major systems—the biological system and the behavioral system (role of medicine to focus on the biological system and role of nursing focus on

the behavioral system. Human being is a behavioral system comprised of subsystems constantly trying to maintain a steady state with patterned, repetitive, and purposeful, ways of behaving that link to him/her to the environment.
- *Health:* Health is the opposite of illness. Health is influenced by biological, psychological and social factors. A lack of balance in the structure or functional requirements of the subsystems lead to poor health. When the system requires a minimal amount of energy for maintenance, a larger supply of energy is available to affect biological process and recovery.
- *Environment:* Environment includes all factors that are not part of a person's behavioral system but has influence of the behavioral system. The nurse can manipulate it to achieve heath for the client. The person is able to continue with successful behaviors if the environment becomes stable.

Concepts of Johnson's Behavior System Model

- *Behavior:* The output of intraorganismic structures and processes as they are coordinated and articulated by and responsive to changes in sensory stimulation. Behavior is affected by the actual or implied presence of others that has been shown to have major adaptive significance.
- *System:* According to her, the system which functions as a whole by virtue of organized independent interaction of its parts.
- *Behavioral system:* Man is a system that indicates the state of the system through behaviors. It consists of patterned, repetitive and purposeful ways of behaving. The system is flexible enough to accommodate the influences affecting it.
- *Subsystem:* Subsystem is a mini system maintained in relationship to the entire system when it or the environment is not disturbed. Behavioral system has to perform many tasks, so the system evolves into subsystem. Each subsystem has to perform specialized tasks. Each subsystem has particular goal and function. Johnson describes seven subsystems that are open, linked and interrelated. The seven subsystems are the following:
  - *Attachment-affiliative subsystem:* Its functions are accomplishment of the security needed for survival as well as social inclusion, intimacy, and the formation and maintenance of strong social bonds. It forms the basis for all social organization.
  - *Dependency subsystem:* Dependency subsystem means behavior designed to get 'approval, attention or recognition and physical assistance'. It helps to enhance behavior that calls for a nurturing response. Developmentally, dependency behavior evolves from almost total dependence on others to a greater degree of dependence on self. Some degree of interdependence is essential for the survival of social groups.

- *Ingestive subsystem:* Its function is to satisfy appetite, with regard to 'when, how, why, how much, and under what conditions the individual eats', which is governed by social and psychological considerations as well as biological requirements for food and fluids.
- *Eliminative subsystem:* Its function is elimination, with regard to 'when, how, and under what conditions the individual eliminates waste.' Behaviors for excretion of waste is vary according to the culture.
- *Sexual subsystem:* Its functions are both procreation and gratification, with regard to behaviors dependent upon the individual's biological sex, including, but not limited to, courting and mating. This response system begins with the development of gender role identity and includes sex-role behaviors also.
- *Achievement subsystem:* Its function is mastery or control of some aspect of self or environment, with regard to intellectual, physical, mechanical, creative, social, and care-taking skills.
- *Aggressive subsystem:* Its function is protection and preservation of self and society. The individual and their property should be respected and protected:
  - *Drive or goal, set, choice, and action or behavior* is four elements of the structure of each subsystem.
  - Motivation for behavior is the *drive or goal.* The specific drive of each subsystem cannot be directly observed but must be inferred from the individual's actual behavior and from the consequences of that behavior.
  - *Set* defined as the individual's predisposition to act in certain ways, rather than in other ways, to fulfill the function of the subsystem. It is also inferred from observed behavior.
  - *Choice* defined as the individual's total behavior repertoire for fulfilling subsystem functions. The behavioral repertoire encompasses the scope of action alternatives from which the person can choose.
  - *Action or behavior* defined as the actual behavior in a situation and is the only structural element that can be observed directly.

- *Equilibrium:* According to her equilibrium is defined as 'a stabilized but more or less transitory, resting state in which the individual is in harmony with himself and with his environment. It implies that biological and other and with impinging social forces. It is not synonymous with a state of health, since it may be found either in health or illness'.
- *Tension:* According to Johnson tension means the system's adjustment to demands, change or growth, or to actual disruptions. It is the end product of the disturbance in equilibrium.
- *Stressor:* A stimulus from the internal or external environment that results in stress or instability. Stimuli may be positive or negative.
- *Structure:* It means the parts of the system that make up the whole.

Attachment and affiliation
Dependency
Elimination
Behavioral disorder
Forces and stress
Sexuality
Ingestion
Aggression
Achievements
Effective functions and adaptations
Ineffective

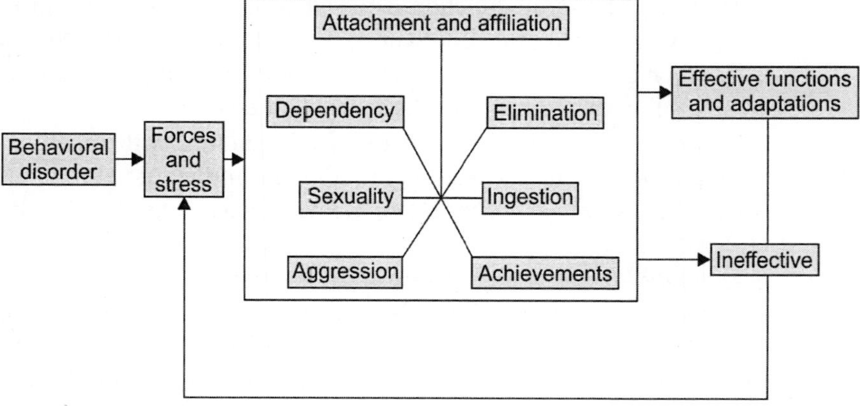

Fig. 5.1: Johnson behavior system model

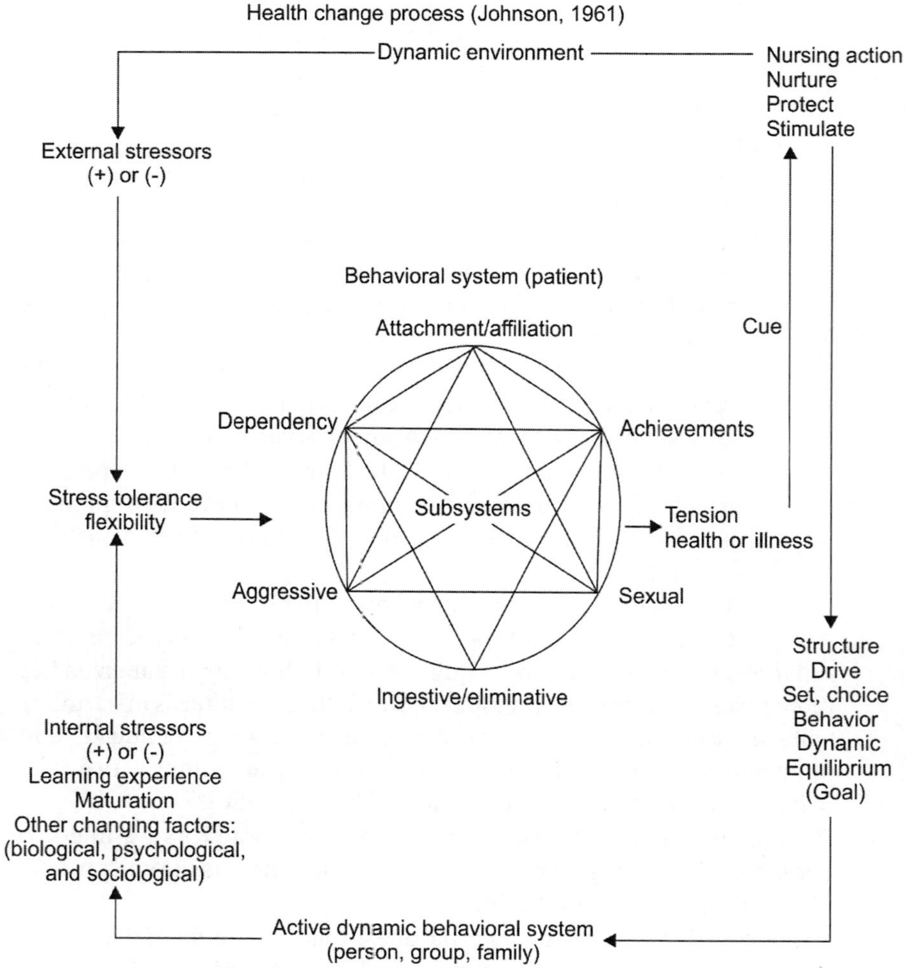

Health change process (Johnson, 1961)
Dynamic environment
Nursing action
Nurture
Protect
Stimulate
External stressors
(+) or (-)
Behavioral system (patient)
Attachment/affiliation
Cue
Dependency
Achievements
Stress tolerance
flexibility
Subsystems
Tension
health or illness
Aggressive
Sexual
Ingestive/eliminative
Structure
Drive
Set, choice
Behavior
Dynamic
Equilibrium
(Goal)
Internal stressors
(+) or (-)
Learning experience
Maturation
Other changing factors:
(biological, psychological,
and sociological)
Active dynamic behavioral system
(person, group, family)

Fig. 5.2: Johnson seven behavioral subsystem

Assumptions of the Theory

- **Assumptions are divided into three categories. They are:**
  - Assumptions about system
  - Assumption about structure
  - Assumption about functions.
- **Assumptions about the systems in the model:**
  - Firstly, there is 'organization, interaction, interdependency and integration of the parts and elements of behaviors that go to make up the subsystem.'
  - Secondly, 'a system tends to achieve a balance among the various forces operating within and upon it and that man strive continually to maintain a behavioral system balance and steady state by more or less automatic adjustments and adaptations to the natural forces impinging upon him.'
  - Thirdly, a behavioral system which requires and results in some degree of regularity and consistency in behavior, it is essential to individual as it is functionally significant as an individual and in social life.
  - Lastly, systems balance reflects adjustments and adaptations that are successful to some degree.
- **Assumptions about the structure:**
  - From the form the behavior takes and the consequence it achieves can be inferred what '*Drive*' has been stimulated and what '*Goal*' is being sought.
  - Each person has a predisposition to act with reference to the goal, in certain ways rather than the other. This predisposition is known as '*SET*.'
  - Each subsystem has a repertoire of choice known as '*Scope of Action*.'
  - Lastly, assumption is that it produce 'observable outcome' that is the individual's behavior.
- **Assumptions about the functions:** Each subsystem has three functional requirements:
  - The system must be '*protected*' from toxic influences with which the system cannot cope.
  - Each system should be '*nurtured*' through the input of appropriate supplies from the environment.
  - The system must be '*stimulated*' for use to augment growth and prevent stagnation.

Nursing Process

- *Assessment:* Grubbs developed an assessment tool based on Johnson's seven subsystems. She added a subsystem known as restorative. An assessment based on behavioral model does not easily allow the nurse to gather detailed information about the biological systems: the eight subsystem include:

1. *Affiliation:* Focus on presence of significant others.
2. *Dependency:* Significant others in the society will help the individual to meet those need which is he/she need to meet.
3. *Sexuality:* Focus on sexual pattern and behavior.
4. *Aggression:* Means how individual protect themselves from perceived threats for safety.
5. *Elimination:* Patterns of defecation and urination and social context in which the pattern occurs.
6. *Ingestion:* Patterns of food and fluid intake and social context in which the patterns occurs.
7. *Achievement:* Means how the individual changes the environment to achieve of goals.
8. *Restorative:* Which focused on activities of daily living.

- *Diagnosis:* Diagnosis tends to be general to the system than specific to the problem. In Johnson model, she not wrote about the nursing diagnosis. Grubb has developed four categories of nursing diagnosis from Johnson's behavioral system model. They are the following:
  1. *Insufficiency:* As a state which exists when a subsystem is not functioning or developed to its fullest capacity because of lack of adequacy and functional requirements.
  2. *Discrepancy:* Behavior that does not meet the goal.
  3. *Incompatibility:* Behavior of two subsystem conflict in the same situation with each other to the loss of the individual.
  4. *Dominance:* Behavior of the one subsystem is used more than the other subsystem.
- *Planning:* Clients input into the plan is less because of that implementation of the nursing care related to the diagnosis may be difficult. The plan will focus on nurses actions to change clients behavior, these plan then have a goal, to bring about homeostasis in a subsystem, based on nursing assessment of the individuals drive, set, behavior, repertoire, and observable behavior. The plan includes protection, nurturance or stimulation of the identified subsystem.
- *Implementation:* Main focus on the equilibrium of the individual through the nurses' action.
- *Evaluation:* Evaluation is based on the achievement of a goal of balance in the identified subsystems. The nurse may have goal for the individual to return to the baseline behavior, if the baseline data of the individual are available. The nurse should be able to observe the return to the previous behavior patterns, if the alterations in the behavior that are planned to occur. Johnson's behavioral model with the nursing process is a nurse centered activity, with the nurse determining the client's needs and state behavior appropriate for that need.

Characteristics of a Theory

- Interrelate concepts to create a different way of viewing a phenomenon: Concepts of Johnson's theory are interrelated.
- Theories must be logical in nature—this theory is logical in nature.
- Theories must be simple yet generalizable—Johnson's theory is simple.
- Theories can be bases of hypothesis that can be tested—many research studies are conducted applying Johnson's theory.
- Theories contribute to and assist in increasing the body of knowledge within the discipline through the research implemented to validate them.
- Theories can be utilized by practitioners to guide and improve their practice.
- Theories must be consistent with other validated theories, laws and principles but will leave unanswered questions that need to be investigated.

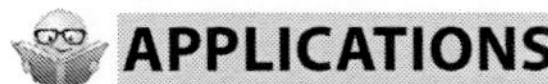

APPLICATIONS

Nursing Education

- This theory can be used in research and education.
- Loveland and Wilkerson concluded that this model has utility in nursing education by analyzing it.
- Person as a behavioral system has goals and straight forward course planning and can be used in curriculum.
- The individual is observed as a whole considering external influences, and studied within the subsystems.
- The nursing processes linked with theoretical models are commonly used to address all areas.

Nursing Administration

- The cooperation of staff is needed, to implement Dorothy Johnson's theory.
- Social workers will be needed for environmental issues and also for economic issues that affect medication fulfillment.
- This theory has been used for administration as a framework when making decisions concerning the management of impaired nurses.

Nursing Research

- According to her, nursing research need to identify and explain behavioral system disorder which arise in connection with illness and develop the rationale for the management.
- Many nursing researchers have demonstrated the Johnson's model is useful in practice.

Nursing Practice

- Within the Behavioral System Theory 'both deductive and inductive systems thinking is evident.'
- The 'system' as a whole works well. But when broken down, looses it's synergistic effect.
- Understanding of the Theory must progress from the bigger picture, or 'whole,' to the individual parts.
- The conceptual model provides a diagnostic and treatment orientation to the practice.
- 'Johnson also believed that groups of individuals could be considered groups of interactive behavioral systems.'
- Grice (1997) used Johnson's model and found that the nurse, patient, and situational characteristics influenced assessment and administration of antianxiety decision-making and antipsychotic medication for psychiatric patient admitted at certain hours.

Limitation

- Johnson in her behavioral system model does not clearly interrelate her concepts of subsystems.
- The concepts are difficult to use because definition of concept is so abstract.
- It is difficult to test Johnson's model by development of hypothesis.
- The focus on the behavioral system makes it difficult for nurses to work with physically impaired individual to use this theory.
- The model is given importance to individual so the nurses working with the group have difficulty in its implementation.
- The model is given importance to individual not to the family.
- Johnson does not define the expected outcomes when one of the system is affected by the nursing implementation an implied expectation is made that all human in all cultures will attain same outcome—homeostasis.
- Johnson's model is not flexible.

Critiquing the Theory

- *Clarity*: The structure of Dorothy Johnson's theory is clear. The relationships have been clearly stated.
- *Simplicity*: Theory is complex with many factors that affect each other.
- *Empirical Precision:* This theory is used in many research work has been found testable and applicable in research.
- *Generality:* Her Model is applicable to all human beings from infancy to the elderly. This theory has been applied in different clinical settings.

 PRACTICAL APPLICATION OF JOHNSON'S BEHAVIORAL SYSTEMS MODEL

Mrs Uma, a 50-year-old female was admitted to Emergency department with complains of decrease level of consciousness (LOC), nausea and vomiting. Her Glasgow coma scale score was 12/15, blood pressure 180/90, pulse rate 108, respiratory rate 22 cpm, temperature 99° Fahrenheit and O_2 sat 88%. Blood sugar 450 mg/dl, blurring of vision, dysarthria, and severe right-sided weakness. Mrs Uma and her husband quarrel with each other and Mrs Uma fell down on the ground so she was admitted hospital within 15 minutes. She was immediately sent for CT scan and diagnosed with acute ischemic attack. Mrs Uma transferred to neuro ICU and thrombolytic therapy was immediately started. The nurse started to do the neurological examination. Then she started on her nursing admission process. The daughter of the patient answered her brief interview since the Mrs Uma cannot fully express herself. The daughter told to nurse that her mother was admitted to the hospital a week ago because of acute right-sided weakness and inability to speak. Her past medical history revealed that the medication for her hypertension was not taken properly due to financial problem. Mrs Uma, a graduate who worked in an insurance firm, is married to Mr Pandey. She lives with her husband and four children in their home. Her husband is unemployed, and an alcoholic. Her daughter told me that her father gradually became depressed after he was terminated from his work. Her mother became so occupied with her work in trying to support her four children. Her daughter also told that their family is slowly breaking into pieces.

Sub system	Assessment		Diagnosis	Planning	Implementation	Evaluation
	Subjective	Objective				
Affiliation	'I do not want to see my husband yet'	She changed the topic whenever husband was mentioned	Impaired social interaction related to previous argument with husband as verbalized by patient 'I do not want to see my husband yet'	Gradually introduce husband to her and tell the importance of their relationship. Talk to her husband regarding her condition and include him during nursing care gradually.	Talked to her husband and ask few questions about their relationship Demonstrated her husband how to check her blood sugar	She tells story about her husband

Contd...

Contd...

Sub system	Assessment		Diagnosis	Planning	Implementation	Evaluation
	Subjective	Objective				
Dependency	'I do not need my husband right now'	She changed the topic whenever husband was mentioned	Chronic sorrow related to previous argument with husband as verbalized by patient 'I do not need my husband right now'	Show the importance of having her husband around that time and this will support her. Ask her husband to express love and support towards her	Ask her if her husband can take her blood sugar	She allowed her husband to take her blood sugar by glucometer but she is not looking at him
Sexuality	Not appropriate for this moment.					
Aggression	Please give me sweet drink	She shows sign of strong desire to have something to eat that is sweet	Impaired readiness for enhance nutrition regimen related to inappropriate choice of food as patient says please give me sweet drink	Educate the client the importance of diet modification and the complication of having high blood sugar	Health teachings on diabetes mellitus and its complications done	She carefully listens and show sign of interest
Elimination	I have difficulty in defecating	She is straining during defecation	Impaired bowel elimination related to decrease bowel movement as manifested by straining during defecation	Educate the client on the importance of drinking water eating green leafy vegetables	Give patient small frequent drinking water and include green leafy vegetables in the food	Her straining is reduced

Contd...

Contd...

Sub system	Assessment		Diagnosis	Planning	Implementation	Evaluation
	Subjective	Objective				
Ingestion	Please give me something sweet drink	She shows the sign of strong desire to have something to eat that is sweet	Self-care deficit feeding related to inappropriate choice of food as patient verbalizes please give me something sweet drink	Educate the client the importance of diet modification and the complication of having high blood sugar	Health teachings on Diabetes mellitus and its complications done	She carefully listens and show sign of interest
Achievement	'When I am sad, I cannot help it to eat something just to forget I am sad'	She begging for food that is not allowed like sweet and high cholesterol, unable to finish hospital serve food	Ineffective health maintenance related to emotional stress and depression as patient verbalizes 'when I am sad, I can't help it to eat something just to forget I am sad'	Educate the client the importance of diet modification and the complication of having high blood sugar and high cholesterol	Health teachings on diabetes mellitus and its complications done	She listens carefully and show sign of interest
Restorative	'I do not think I can return to my usual way of living and to do my daily living activities'	She shows facial expression of hopelessness	Hopelessness related to emotional stress as patient verbalizes 'I do not think I can return to my usual way of living and to do my daily living activities'	Give positive reinforcement and motivation to live like and talking about her children	Health teachings on diabetes mellitus and its complications done and show the result and benefits of having blood sugar monitor and maintain to prevent complications	She listens carefully and show facial expression of interest

CONCLUSION

Johnson's Behavioral System Model could help to guide the future of nursing theories, models, research, and education. By focusing on behavioral rather than biology, this theory differentiates nursing from medicine. In order to focus on the holistic idea of nursing, it is important to think of the behavioral and biological together as health.

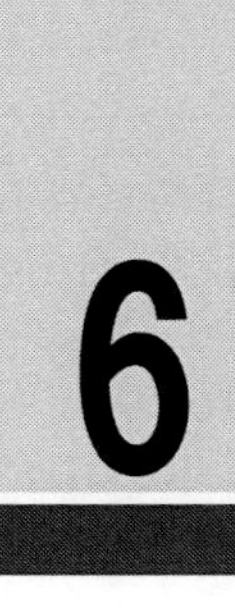

6 Imogene King: Theory of Goal Attainment

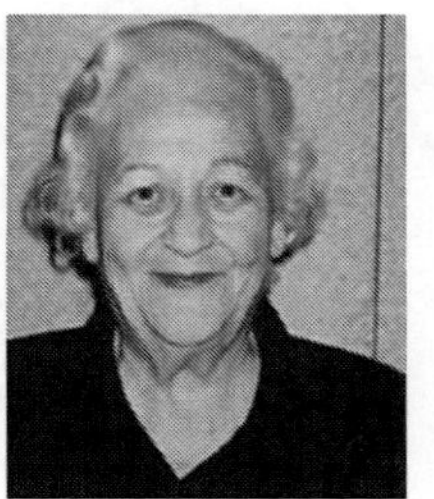

'A professional nurse, with special knowledge and skills, and a client in need of nursing, with knowledge of self and perception of personal problems, meet as strangers in natural environment. They interact mutually, identify problems, establish and achieve goals.'

–Imogene King

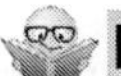 INTRODUCTION

In the early 1960s, Imogene King developed the Theory of Goal Attainment. From the title itself, the model focuses on the achievement of certain life goals. This theory describes that the nurse and client go hand-in-hand in communicating information, set goals together, and then take actions to attain those goals. Imogene M King's Theory of Goal Attainment mainly focus on this process to guide and direct nurses in the nurse-patient relationship, going hand-in-hand with their clients to meet the goals towards good health.

Biography and Achievements

- Imogene King was born on January 30, 1923 in West Point, Iowa. She was the youngest of three children.
- She earned her diploma in nursing education from St. John's Hospital of Nursing in St Louis Missouri in 1945.
- She worked as office nurse, staff nurse, school nurse, and private duty nurse to support herself while studying for a baccalaureate degree.
- She completed her Bachelor of Science in Nursing from St. Louis University in 1948.
- She earned her Masters of Science in Nursing from St. Louis University in 1957.
- She received her Doctorate in Education from Teacher's college, Columbia University, New York in 1961.
- She was an Associate Professor of Nursing from 1961–1966.
- She spent in the academic settings of Ohio State, University, Loyola University, and the University of South Florida from 1966 to 1968.
- Her first theory article appeared in 1964 in a journal edited by Dr Martha Rogers titled *Nursing Science.*

- She was the Director of the School of Nursing at The Ohio State University in Columbus from 1968 to 1972. While at Ohio State, her book *Toward a Theory for Nursing* was published.
- She formulated this theory while she was an Associate Professor of Nursing at Loyola University in Chicago.
- She died because of stroke on December 24, 2007.

ASSUMPTIONS

Explicit Assumptions

- The central focus of nursing is the interaction of person and environment, with the goal being healthy for person.
- Human being is social, sentient, rational, reacting, perceiving, controlling, purposeful, action-oriented, and time-oriented being.
- The interaction process is influenced by perceptions, goals, needs, and values of both the patient and the nurse.
- Individual as a patients have rights to get information, to participate in decisions that may influence their life, health, and society services, and to accept or reject care.
- It is the responsibility of health care members to inform persons of all aspects of health care to help them in making 'informed decision.'
- Incongruities may exist between the goals of health for caregivers and recipients. Individual has the right to either accept or reject any aspect of health care.

Implicit Assumptions

- In the care process clients want to participate actively.
- Clients are conscious, active, and cognitively capable to participate in decision-making.

CONCEPTS AND COMPONENTS OF THE OPEN SYSTEM FRAMEWORK

Imogene King used a **'systems'** approach in the development of her dynamic interacting systems framework and in her subsequent Goal Attainment Theory. She developed a general systems framework and a theory of goal attainment where the framework refers to the three interacting systems—individual or personal system, group or interpersonal system, and society or social system, while the theory of goal attainment pertains to the importance of interaction, perception, communication, transaction, self, role, stress, growth and development, time, and personal space. King emphasizes that both the nurse and the patient bring important knowledge and information to the relationship and that they work together to attain goals.

- *Personal systems (individuals):* The basic elements in the system are the concepts of perception, self, growth and development, body image, learning time, personal space, and coping:
  - *Perception:* Individual's representation of reality and it is unique to each person 'process of organizing interpreting and transforming information from sense data and memory.' It influences all behavior.
  - *Self:* The individual's subjective environment, values, ideas, attitudes, and commitment. It is the composite of thoughts and feelings and which constitute an individual's awareness of his/her individual existence, his/her conception of who and what he/she is.
  - *Growth and Development:* It is the processes that take place in a person's life that help the person move from potential capacity for achievement to self-actualization. The characteristics of growth and development include cellular, molecular and behavioral changes in a person.
  - *Body Image:* The way of an individual perceives his body and the reaction of others to his appearance. Body image is subjective and changes as the individual changes physically or emotionally. It is the part of each stage of growth and development.
  - *Personal space:* It is existing in all directions and is the same everywhere. It is the immediate environment in which nurse and patient interact.
  - *Time:* It is the duration between the occurrence of one event and occurrence of another event. It is defined as a sequence of events moving onwards to the future.
  - *Learning:* It is a process of sensory perception, conceptualization, and critical thinking involving multiple experiences in which changes in concepts, skills, symbols, habit and values can be evaluated in observable behaviors.
  - *Coping:* It is constantly changing cognitive and behavioral efforts to manage specific external and internal demands that are appraised as taxing the resources.
- **Interpersonal systems (group): (Dyadic or triadic or small group):** When personal systems come in contact with one another and form interpersonal system. It is formed by the human beings interaction. Two interacting individual form a dyad, three form a triad, and four or more form small or large groups. It requires an understanding of the concepts of communication, interaction, role, stress/stressors and transaction:
  - *Interaction:* It is the acts of two or more persons in mutual presence. It is the process of perception and communication between individual and environment and between individual and individual, represented by verbal nonverbal behavior that is goal oriented. Each person's interaction is unique which brings different knowledge, needs, goals, perception, past experience and perceptions which influence the interaction.

- *Communication:* It is the information processing, a change of information from one individual to another. Communication may be either direct or indirect.
- *Transaction:* It is the process of interaction between an individual and another individual or an individual and the environment to attain goals that are valued.
- *Role:* Role means set of behaviors expected when occupying a position in social system. The elements of role are follows:
  - Role consists of a set of expected behavior of those who occupy a position in a social system.
  - Role consists of a set of procedure or rules that define the obligations and rights associated with a position in an organization.
  - Role is a relationship of two or more individual who are interacting for a purpose in a particular situation.
- *Stress:* Stress is a dynamic state whereby an individual interacts with the environment to maintain balance for growth, development and performance which involves an exchange of energy and information between the individual and the environment for regulation and control stressors.

• *Social Systems:* Social systems form when interpersonal systems come together to form larger systems; such as families, religious groups, school, work, and peer groups. The social systems are consist of social roles, behaviors, and practices that are developed to maintain values and include organizations, authority, power, status, and decision-making:
- *Organization:* A system whose continuous activities are conducted to attain goals. King proposes four parameters for organization:
  a. Human values, behavior patterns, needs, goals, and expectations.
  b. A natural environment in which material and human resources are essential for attaining goals.
  c. Employers and employees, or parents, and children, who form groups that collectively interact to attain goals.
  d. Technology that facilitate goal achievement.
- *Authority:* It is the power or the person who make decisions that guide other person's actions.
- *Power:* It is the capacity to use resources in organizations to attain goal.
- *Status:* It is the position of a person in a group or a group in relation to other groups in an organization.
- *Decision-making:* Dynamic and systematic process by which a goal directed choice of perceived alternatives is made and acted upon by persons or groups to attain a goal.
- *Control:* It is added as a sub-concept in the social system.

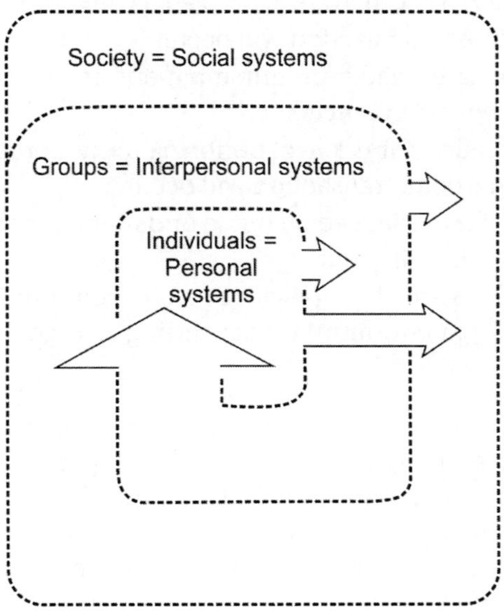

Fig. 6.1: Dynamic interacting systems

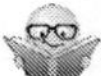 THEORY OF GOAL ATTAINMENT

King has been derived this theory from her open system framework. This theory derived from the conceptual framework organizes elements in the process of nurse-patient interactions that result in outcomes, that is goal achievement. Among the three systems, the conceptual framework of interpersonal system had the greatest influence on the development of King's theory. She stated that 'Although personal systems and social systems influence quality of care, the major elements in a theory of goal attainment are discovered in the interpersonal systems in which two people, who are usually strangers, come together in a health care organization to help and to be helped to maintain a state of health that permits functioning in roles':

- This theory describes a dynamic, interpersonal relationship in which an individual grows and develops to achieve certain life goals.
- The concepts of theory are interaction, perception, communication, transaction, self, role, stress, growth and development, time, and personal space. These concepts are interrelated in every nursing situation. Refer above for definition these terms.
- Factors which affect the achievement of goal are: roles, stress, space and time.

King developed predictive propositions from the theory of goal attainment, which includes

- If perceptual interaction accuracy is present in nurse-patient interactions, transaction will occur.

- If nurse and patient make transaction, goal will be achieved.
- If goal are attained, satisfaction will occur.
- If transactions are made in nurse-patient interactions, growth and development will be enhanced.
- If role of expectations and role of performance as perceived by nurse and patient are congruent, transaction will occur.
- If role conflict is experienced by nurse or patient or both, stress in nurse-patient interaction will occur.
- If nurse with special knowledge skill communicate appropriate information to patient, mutual goal setting and goal achievement will occur.

Each person involved in an interaction brings different ideas, attitudes, and perception to exchange. The people come together for a purpose and perceive each other; each makes a judgment and takes mental action or decides to act. Then each reacts to the other and the situation (perception, judgment, action, and reaction). According to King only interaction and transaction are observable.

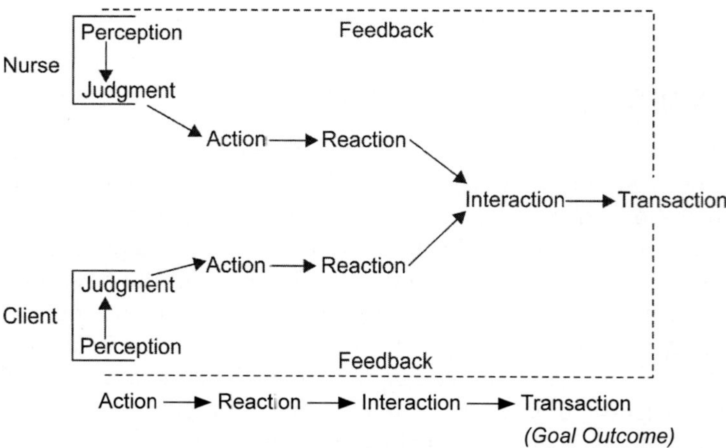

Fig. 6.2: A human interaction process

METAPARADIGM

Human Being/Person

- Person is a social being who are rational and sentient.
- The three fundamental needs of person are the following:
  a. The need for the health information that is unable at the time when it is needed and can be used
  b. The need for care that seek to prevent illness
  c. The need for care when person are unable to help themselves.

- She proposes three basic premises; human being is:
  a. **Man is a reactive being:**
     - Human being is aware of other things; persons and events in the environment.
     - At various times this awareness makes the being respond to the environment based upon his perceptions, expectations and needs.
  b. **Man as a time oriented being:**
     - Human being is influenced by time orientation.
     - Each man presents with by his/her past experience that influences his/her actions.
     - His/her awareness of the present helps shape the future.
  c. **Man as a social being:**
     - Man has a continuous exchange with individual in the environment.
     - Language is a social link for persons and facilitates interpersonal communication.
- King identifies seven other characteristics of individual:
  a. The ability to perceive—these perceptions will influence behavior and thus life and health.
  b. The ability to think—thinking is based upon the inquiring mind of person. When person thinks he/she has the ability to discriminate and identify relationships.
  c. The ability to feel or to have emotions about the environment.
  d. The ability to choose between alternative courses of action.
  e. The ability to set goals.
  f. The ability to select means to attain the goals.
  g. The ability to make decisions dependent on other characteristics.

Environment

- King used the terms environment, health care environment, internal environment, external environment.
- Environment is the background for human interactions.
- Internal environment of individual transforms energy to enable them to adjust to continue external environmental changes.
- External environment involves formal and informal organizations. Nurse is a part of the client's environment.
- The person continuously adjusts to stressors in the internal and external environment.
- Environment is a function of balance between internal and external actions.

Health

- Health is a dynamic life experience of man, which implies continuous adjustment to stressors in the internal and external environment through

optimum use of one's resources to achieve maximum potential for daily living.
- King also defined health as an ability to function in social roles.
- King describes health as a dynamic state of a person in which change is a constant and ongoing process.
- She defined illness as 'a deviation from normal, that, an imbalance in an individual's biological structure or in his psychological make-up, or a conflict in an individual's social relationships.'
- In King's definition of health there is no consideration of age group or point of time.

Nursing

- According to King Nursing is a process of actions, reaction, interaction, and transaction whereby nurses assist people of any age and socioeconomic group to meet their basic needs in performing activities of daily living and to cope with health and illness at some particular point in the life cycle.
- The *domain of nursing* includes promotion of health, maintenance and restoration of health, care of the sick and injured and care of the dying.
- King also defined nursing as a helping profession that 'provides a service to meet a social need.'
- As a *goal of nursing* is to help people and groups attain, maintain, and restore health so they can function in their roles.
- Function of professional nurse to interpret information in nursing process to plan, implement and evaluate nursing care.
- Nurses are key figures in health care delivery as partners with physicians, social workers, and allied health professionals in enhancing health, in preventing disease, and in managing client care.

Theory of Goal Attainment and Nursing Process

King describes the nursing process as 'a dynamic, ongoing interpersonal process in which the nurse and the patient are viewed as a system with each affecting the behavior of the other and both being affected by factors within the situation.'

The three-dimensional nursing process based on King's Theory. The nursing process is elaborated through the Theory of Goal Attainment. (*See Flowchart on next page*)

- King began to refer to the nursing process discussed by the theory as an 'interaction-transaction process model.'
- The components of the nursing process, or transactional model, where identified as perception, judgment, action, reaction, disturbance, mutual goal setting, exploration of means to achieve the goal, agreement on means to achieved goal, transaction, and attainment of the goal.

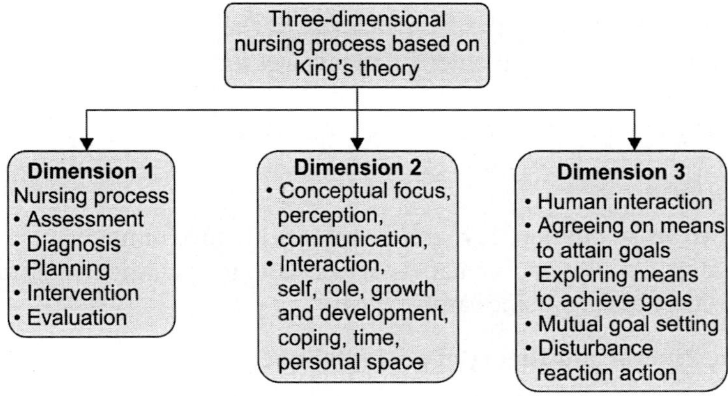

Fig. 6.3: Three-dimensional nursing process based on King's theory

Assessment

- During interaction with the client assessment done by the nurse.
- In this phase the nurse and the patient perceive each other, make mental judgments about the other, take some mental action, react to each one's perception of the other, communicate, and begin to interact.
- The nurse brings special knowledge and skills and patient brings knowledge of self and perception of problems of concern, to this interaction.
- During assessment nurse collects data regarding patient (patient's perception of self, growth and development, and current health status, roles, etc.)
- Communication is required to verify accuracy of perception, for interaction and transaction.
- Perception is the base for collection and interpretation of data.

Nursing Diagnosis

- To make nursing diagnosis in nursing process the data collected by assessment are used.
- In process of achieving goal the nurse identifies the problems, concerns and disturbances about which individual seek help.

Planning

- Planning for interventions to solve those problems is done after diagnosis.
- In this phase, interaction can be observed directly, and the data about those interactions can be recorded.
- In goal achievement planning is represented by setting goals and making decisions about and being agreed on the means to attain goals.
- This part of transaction and patient's participation is encouraged in making decision on the means to attain the goals.

Implementations

- In nursing process implementation involves the actual activities to attain the goals.
- In goal attainment it is the continuation of transaction.

Evaluation

- It involves to finding out whether goals are attained or not.
- In king description evaluation speaks about attainment of goal and effectiveness of nursing care.

Nursing Process and Theory of Goal Attainment

Nursing process method	Nursing process theory
A system of oriented actions	A system of oriented concepts
Assessment	Perception, communication and interaction of nurse and patient
Planning	• Decision-making about the goals • Be agree on the means to attain the goals
Implementation	Transaction made
Evaluation	Goal attained

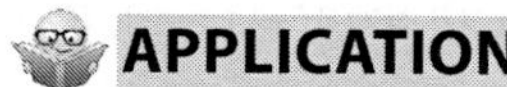

APPLICATION

Practice

- The theory's relationship to practice is obvious because the profession of nursing functions through persons and groups within the environment.
- Useful in individualized plans of care while encouraging active participation from patient's in decision-making.
- Coker and Schreiber (1990) used this model for bedside nursing practice in the hospital setting.
- Hampton (1994) also used this model for managing care program in hospital settings.

Education

- This model has been used for curriculum design in nursing programs and framework for books.
- It provides a systematic means of viewing the nursing profession, organizing a body of knowledge for nursing, and clarifying nursing as a discipline.
- In Ohio State University School of Nursing used this framework for the baccalaureate program.

Research

- Research can be designed and conducted to implement this system in a hospital unit, in ambulatory care, in community nursing, and home care.
- Rooda (1992) used this model for Multicultural Nursing Practice.

Limitations

- It lacks clear definition of environment.
- This theory is limited in settings in regard to natural environment.
- Mutuality between nurse and client is must for goal attainment.
- Repeated definitions of concepts.
- This theory is not a perfect theory.

Critique of the Theory

- *Simplicity:* King's theory has nine major concepts, that make it complex; but easily understood because they are defined to show interrelations in nursing practice.
- *Clarity:* All concepts are clear and conceptually derived from identified characteristics.
- *Generality:* This theory has limited applications in areas of nursing. It is impossible that theory will address every person, event, and situation.
- *Empirical Precision:* Goal attainment could be measured along the effectiveness of nursing care.
- *Derivable Consequences:* This theory deals with choices, alternatives, participation of all persons in decision-making and specifically deals with outcomes of nursing care.

Practical Application of Imogene King: Theory of Goal Attaintment

Mrs Saparna, 29-year-old female underwent appendectomy four days before and she is expecting discharge from hospital.

Nursing Process

1. Assessment	
The first process in nursing process is nurse meets the client and communicates and interacts with her. Assessment is conducted by gathering data about the client-based on relevant concepts.	
Mrs Saparna is 29-year-old married; got admitted hospital on 25/06/15 with a complaint of acute pain in the right lower abdominal pain and diagnosed as appendicitis. She underwent appendectomy on same day. The following areas were addressed for gathering data.	
What is the client's perception of the situation?	She says 'I have undergone surgery for appendicitis'. 'The wound is getting healed, I have no other problem' 'I have pain in the area of surgery when moving' I am taking medicines for diabetes mellitus for the last 5 years from here'

Contd...

Contd...

What are nurse's perceptions of the situation?	Mrs Saparna underwent appendectomy on 25th June. Client is at risk of developing infection. She has pain related to surgical incision. Patient may develop diabetes mellitus related complications in future.
What other information does the nurse need to assist this client to achieve health?	**History** *Identification details:* Mrs Saparna, 29-year-old married, female, home maker studied up to 10th Standard, a practicing Hindu, got admitted Hospital on 25/06/15 with a complaint right lower abdominal pain and diagnosed as appendicitis. She is underwent appendectomy on same day. *Present history of illness:* 39-weeks of period of gestation and leaking per vagina. She is a known case of diabetes mellitus since 5 years. *Past health history:* She is on treatment for diabetes mellitus. No other significant illness
	Family history: Her mother and father is a known case of diabetes mellitus elder brother also underwent appendectomy 4 years back. *Socioeconomic status:* Middle class status ₹ 150000/- per month. *Life style:* Vegetarian. Nonsmoker or nonalcoholic. She is aware about health care facilities *Physical examination:* Alert, conscious and oriented. Moderately built, adequate nourishment, with BMI of 23. Vital signs-normal General head-to-foot examination reveals normal finding and healing surgical wound. Subjective problems: Pain at the surgical wound site, lack of bowel movement for 3 days. **Review of relevant systems**: *GI system* Inspection: Healing wound, No infection, No redness, No swelling. • Auscultation: Normal bowel sounds • Palpation: No pain at the site, Normal abdominal organs • Percussion: No dull sound suggesting fluid collection or ascites *Genitourinary system* • Inspection: No infection, No swelling or enlargement. • Palpation: No complaint of pain. • Percussion: No fluid collection • Auscultation: Normal Bowel sounds **Laboratory Investigations:** • FBS–120 mg/dl • Na (130–143 mEq/dl)–32 mEq/dl • K^+ (3.5–5 mg/dl)–3.8 mEq/dl • Urea (8–35 mg/dl)–27 mg/dl • Sr. Cr (0.6–1.6 mg/dl)–<1 mg/ dl **Other investigations:** CT scan and USG: Findings are normal

Contd...

Contd...

What does this information means to this situation?	• She has acute pain at the site of surgical wound. • She has family history of Appendectomy. • Client has risk for infection due to inadequate knowledge. • She is at risk of developing complications of diabetes mellitus. • She needs education regarding health maintenance.
What conclusion (judgment) does this client make?	• She requires management for her pain on surgical area. • She understands the need taking care of health risks and agrees to work on these aspects.
What conclusion (judgment) does this client make?	Based on the assessment following nursing diagnoses were formulated, i.e. the clinical judgment about the client's actual and potential problems.
Nursing diagnosis The data collected by assessment are used to make nursing diagnosis in nursing process.	• Acute pain related to surgical incision. • Risk for infection related to surgical incision. • Risk for constipation related to bed rest, pain medication and NPO or soft diet.
According to King in process of attaining goal, the nurse identifies the problems, concerns and disturbances about which individual seek help	• Deficient knowledge regarding the treatment and home care. • Ineffective health maintenance.

2. Planning	
Identifying the goals and planning to achieve these goals (this step is congruent with planning in the traditional nursing process)	
What goals does the nurse think will serve the client's best interest?	• The patient will experience improved comfort, as evidenced by: – A decrease in the rating of the pain, – The ability to rest and sleep comfortably • The patient will be free of infection as evidenced by normal temperature, normal vital signs. • The patient will have improved bowel elimination, as evidenced by: – Elimination of stool without straining • Patient will acquire adequate knowledge regarding the treatment and home care. • Patient will attend to health problems promptly.
What are the client's goals?	Client's goals are: • Freedom from pain • Rapid healing • Adequate bowel movement • Acquiring adequate knowledge regarding his health problems

Contd...

Contd...

Are the client's goals and professional goals are congruent?	Yes
What are the priority goals?	Relief of pain: • Freedom from infection • Adequate bowel movement • Improvement knowledge aspect of health conditions • Prompt attendance to health problems
What does the client perceives as the best way to attain goals?	• Working with the health professionals • Gaining knowledge • Disclosing adequate information regarding health problems
Is the client willing to work towards the goals?	Yes
What does the nurse perceive to be the best way to achieve the goals?	**Goal 1:** • Assess the characteristics of pain • Administration of prescribed medicine • Monitor the responses to drug therapy • Provide calm, efficient manner that reassures the client and minimizes anxiety • Provide a comfortable position as per her requests.
	Goal 2: • Monitor vital signs • **Administer antibiotics as advised** • **Use aseptic techniques while** changing dressing • **Kept the surgical wound site clean** • **Report surgeon regarding early signs of infection** **Goal 3:** • Ensure that the patient has adequate bulk in diet and adequate fluid intake • Instruct the patient on prevention of straining and avoiding valsalva maneuvers • Consult treating physician regarding medications. **Goal 4:** • Explain the treatment measures to the client and their benefits in a simple understandable language. • Explain demonstrate about the home care. • Clarify the doubts of the client as the client may present with some matters of importance. • Repeat the information whenever necessary to reinforce learning. **Goal 5:** Health education given about the following: • Restriction of heavy weight lifting (more than 20 kg) for 6 months • Further management which may be necessary • Diet control for his diabetes mellitus • Rehabilitation measures to promote better living.

Contd...

Contd...

Are the goals short-term or long- term?	Goals are both short-term and long-term.
What modifications required based on mutuality?	• Pain is tolerable to the client and requires no SOS medication • Constipation is not that severe enough to take medication • Other interventions are mutually acceptable.

3. Implementation	
Is the nurse doing what the client and nurse has agreed upon?	Yes
How is the nurse carrying out the actions?	On a mutually acceptable manner in accordance with the goals set.
When does the nurse carry out the action?	According to priority, a few interventions require immediate attention. Other interventions are carried out during the period of hospitalization.
Why is the nurse carrying out the action?	Client's condition demands nursing care.
Is it reasonable to think that the identified goals will be reached by carrying out the action?	Yes

4. Evaluation	
Are nurse's actions helping the client to attain mutually defined goals?	Yes
How well are goals being met?	• Short-term goals are met before discharge from hospital • Long-term goals are expected to be met, because the client is motivated to continue home care.
What is client's response to nurse's actions?	Client is satisfied with nurse's actions
Are other factors hindering goal achievement?	No
How should the plan be changed to achieve goals?	• Health teaching can be modified according to developmental stage. • Involvement of family member in care of the Client.

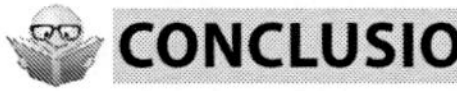

CONCLUSION

Imogene king derived a theory of goal attainment from her open system framework. This theory is based on a philosophy of individuals and open systems framework. This theory is useful, testable and applicable to nursing practice. King contributed to the advancement of nursing knowledge through the development of her conceptual system and middle-range Theory of Goal Attainment. By focusing on the attainment of goals, or outcomes, by nurse-client relationships, King provided a conceptual system and middle-range theory that has demonstrated its usefulness to nurses. Nurses working in a variety of settings with clients from around the world continue to use King's work to improve the quality of client care.

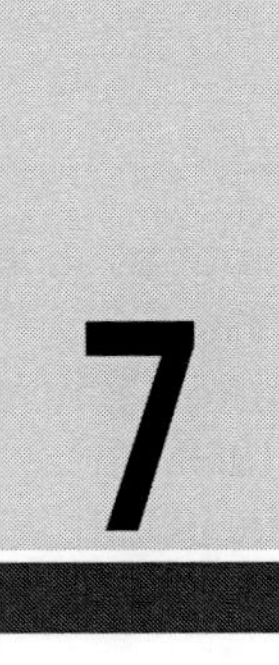

7 Myra Levine: Conservation Model

'Ethical behavior is not the display of one's moral rectitude in times of crisis; it is the day-to-day expression of one's commitment to other persons and ways in which human beings relate to one another in their daily interactions.'

–Myra Levine (1972)

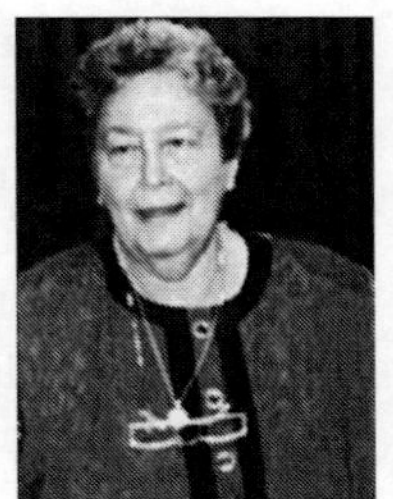

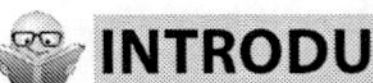

INTRODUCTION

Florence Nightingale taught that nursing theories describe and explain that what is not nursing. Today, knowledge development in nursing is taking place on several fronts, with a variety of scholarly approaches contributing to advance in the discipline. Nursing practice increasingly take place in interdisciplinary community settings, and the form of nursing in acute care of settings which is rapidly changing various paradigms and value. Systems that express perspectives held by several groups within discipline ground the knowledge and practice of nursing.

BIOGRAPHY

Myra Estrin Levine (1920–1996) has been called a Renaissance women-highly principled, remarkable, and committed to what happens to patient's quality of life.

She was born in Chicago, Illinois. She was the oldest of three children. She had one sister and one brother. Levine developed an interest in nursing because of her father who was frequently ill and required nursing care due to gastrointestinal (GI) problems.

Educational Achievements

- Levine received her diploma from Cook Country School of Nursing in 1944.
- She received her Bachelor of Science degree from the University of Chicago in 1949.
- After graduation, she worked as a private duty nurse, civilian nurse for the US army, surgical nursing supervisor, and also in nursing administration.
- Levine received her Master of Science in Nursing from Wayne State University in 1962.

- Following masters, she taught nursing at many different institutions such as University of Illinois at Chicago and Tel Aviv University in Israel.
- She published 77 articles which included 'An Introduction to Clinical Nursing' with multiple publication years on 1969, 1973 and 1989.
- She received an honorary doctorate from Loyola University in 1992.
- She had clinical experience in the operating room and in Oncology Nursing.
- She was a civilian nurse at Drexel Home in Chicago, clinical instructor at Bryan memorial Hospital in Lincoln, Nebraska and administrative supervisor at University of Chicago Clinical and Henry Ford Hospital in Michigan.
- She was Chairperson of clinical nursing at Cook Country School of Nursing and a faculty member at Loyola University, Rush University and University of Illinois.
- She was a visiting professor at Tel Aviv University in Israel and Recanati School of School of Nursing at Ben-Gurion University of Negev in Beer Sheva, Israel.
- She was professor emeritus in medical-surgical Nursing, University of Chicago, a charter Fellow of the American Association of Nurses (FAAN).
- She was a member of Sigma Theta Tau International, from which she received the Elizabeth Russell Belford Award as distinguished educator.

Concepts of Conservational Model

- The major *goal* or *focus* of the conservation model is to promote adaptation and maintain wholeness using the principles of conservation.
- This model guides the nurse to focus on the influence and response at the *organismic level.*
- The nurses can accomplish the goal of the model through the *conservation of energy, structure integrity, personal integrity* and *social integrity.*
- Although *conservation* is focused on outcomes expected when this model is used, she also discussed two other concepts critical to the use of her model, i.e. *adaptation* and *wholeness.*

Adaptation

- Adaptation is the process of change and conservation is the outcome of adaptation.
- Adaptation is the process by which the patient maintains integrity within the realities of the environment.
- Adaptation is achieved through the 'frugal, economic, contained and controlled use of environmental resources by the individual in his or her best interest.'
- Each individual has a unique range of adaptive response. These responses will vary based on heredity, age, gender, or challenges of an illness experience.

For example, the response to weakness of cardiac muscle is an increased heart rate, dilation of the ventricle, and thickening of the myocardial muscle while the response are the same, the timing and manifestation of the organismic response (e.g. pulse rate) will be unique for individual.

Wholeness

- Wholeness is based on Erickson's statement, i.e. wholeness as an open system. 'Wholeness emphasizes a sound, organic, progressive mutually between diversified function and parts within an entirety, the boundaries of which are open and fluid.'
- Levine stated that 'the unceasing interaction of the individual organism with its environment does represent an 'open and fluid' system, and a condition of health, wholeness, exists when the interactions, or constant adaptations to the environment, permit ease—the assurance of integrity... in all the dimensions of life.' This continuous dynamic, open interaction between the internal and external environment provides the basis for holistic thought, the view of the *individual as whole not just an illness.*

Conservation

- Conservation is the product of adaptation.
- Conservation is derived from the Latin word *conservation,* meaning 'to keep together.'
- 'Conservation describes the way that complex systems are able to continue to function even when severely challenged.'
- Through conservation, individuals are able to overcome obstacles, adapt accordingly, and will maintain their uniqueness.
- The primary focus of conservation is keeping together of the wholeness of the individual.

PARADIGM OF LEVINE'S THEORY

Levine skillfully weaves her beliefs about human body (person), environment, health and nursing throughout her discussion of conservation and adaptation, as follows:

Human Being (Person)

- Person is who we know out self to be or a sense of identity.
- When a person is being studied, the focus should be on wholeness.
- The person is holistic being who constantly strives to preserve wholeness and integrity.
- The person is also a unique individual in unity and integrity, feeling, believing, thinking and whole system of system.

Environment

- The environment completes the wholeness of the individual.
- The individual has both an *internal* (homeostasis and homeorhesis) and *external* environment (pre-conceptual, operational and conceptual).
  - ***Internal environment:*** The *internal environment* includes both the physiological and pathophysiological aspects of the individual and is constantly challenged by the external environment. The internal environment also combines to the integration of bodily functions that resembles *homeorhesis* rather than *homeostasis* and is subject to challenges the external environment, which always are a form of energy.

    Homeostasis:
    - It is a state of energy sparing that also provides the necessary baselines for a multitude of synchronized physiological and psychological factors.
    - It is also a state of conservation.

    Homeorhesis:
    - Homeorhesis means stabilized flow rather than a static state.
    - It emphasis the fluidity of change within a space-time continuum.
    - It describe the pattern of adaptation, which permit the individual's body to sustain its well-being with the vast changes which encroach upon it from the environment.
  - ***External environment:*** External environment is divided into the pre-conceptual, operational, and conceptual environments.
    - *Pre-conceptual environment:* It is that portion of the external environment in which individuals respond to with their sense organs and which includes light, sound, touch, temperature, chemical change that is smelled or tasted, and position sense and balance.
    - *Operational environment:* It is that portion of the external environment which interacts with living tissue even though the individual does not possess sensory organs that can record the presence of these factors and includes all forms of radiation, microorganisms, and pollutants. In other words, these elements may physically affect individuals but are not perceived by the latter.
    - *Conceptual environment:* It is that portion of the external environment that consists of language, ideas, symbols, and concepts and inventions and encompasses the exchange of language, the ability to think and experience emotion, value systems, religious beliefs, ethnic and cultural traditions, and individual psychological patterns that come from life experiences.

Health

- Health and disease are patterns of adaptive change.
- Health is implied to mean unity and integrity and 'is a wholeness and successful adaptation'.

- The goal of nursing is to promote health.
- It is not only the insult or the injury that is repaired but the person himself or herself.
- It is not merely the healing of an afflicted part. It is rather a return to daily activities, selfhood where the encroachment of the disability can be set aside entirely, and the individual is free to pursue once more his or her own interests without constraint.
- Disease is 'unregulated and undisciplined change and must be stopped or death will ensue.'

Nursing

- Nursing involves engaging in 'human interactions.'
- 'Nursing is a profession as well as an academic discipline, always practiced and studied in concern with all of the disciplines that together form the health sciences.'
- The human interaction relying on communication, rooted in the organic dependency of the individual human being in his relationships with other human beings.
- The nurse enters into a partnership of human experience where sharing moments in time—some trivial, some dramatic—leaves its mark forever on each patient.'

Goal of Nursing

- To promote wholeness, realizing that every individual requires a unique and separate cluster of activities.
- The individual integrity is his/her abiding concern and it is the nurse's responsibility to assist him to defend and to seek its realization.
- The goal of nursing is accomplished through the use of the conservation principles: conservation of energy, conservation of structural integrity, conservation of personal integrity, and conservation of social integrity.

Person and Environment

- Adaptation
- Organismic response
- Conservation
- As it was mentioned above, Levine's Conservation Model discussed that the way in which the person and the environment become congruent over time.
- It is the fit of the person with his or her predicament of time and space.
- The specific adaptive responses make conservation possible occur on many levels; molecular, physiologic, emotional, psychological, and social. These responses are based on three factors (Levine, 1989): Historicity, specificity and redundancy.

- **Adaptation**

  Characteristics

  Historicity:

  - Refers to the notion that adaptive responses are partially based on personal and genetic past history.
  - Each individual is made up of a combination of personal and genetic history, and adaptive responses are the result of both.
  - Adaptations are grounded in history and await the challenges to which they respond.

  Specificity:

  - Refers the fact that each system that makes up a human being has unique stimulus-response pathways.
  - Responses are stimulated by specific stressors and are task-oriented.
  - Responses that are stimulated in multiple pathways tend to be synchronized and occur in a cascade of complimentary (or detrimental in some cases) reactions.
  - Individual responses and their adaptive pattern varies on the base of specific genetic structure.

  Redundancy:

  - Redundancy describes the notion that if one system or pathway, is unable to ensure adaptation, then another pathway may be able to take over and complete the job.
  - This may be helpful when the response is corrective (e.g. the use of allergy shots over a lengthy period of time to diminish the effects of severe allergies by gradually desensitizing the immune system).
  - However, redundancy may be detrimental, such as when previously failed responses are re-established (e.g. when autoimmune conditions cause a person's own immune system to attack previously healthy tissue in the body).
  - Safe and fail options available to the individual to ensure continued adaptation.
- ***Organismic response***
  - A change in behavior of an individual during an attempt to adapt the environment is called organismic response.
  - It helps individual to protect and maintain their integrity.

  They are four types:

  1. *Flight or fight:* An instantaneous response to real or imagined threat, most primitive response.
  2. *Inflammatory:* Response intended to provide for structural integrity and the promotion of healing.

3. *Stress:* Response developed over time and influenced by each stressful experience encountered by person.
4. *Perceptual:* Involves gathering information from the environment and converting it into a meaning experience.

Conservational Principle

- The core, or central concept, of Levine's theory is *conservation* (Levine, 1989).
- When a person is in a state of conservation, it means that individual adaptive responses conform change productively, and with the least expenditure of effort, while preserving optimal function and identity.
- Conservation is achieved through successful activation of adaptive pathways and behaviors that are appropriate for the wide range of responses required by functioning human beings.
- Myra Levine described the *Four Conservation Principles.* These principles focus on conserving an individual's wholeness.
- She described that nursing is a human interaction and proposed four conservation principles of nursing which are concerned with the unity and integrity of individuals. Her framework includes: *Energy, structural integrity, personal integrity, and social integrity.*

  I. ***Conservation of energy***: Refers to balancing energy input and output to avoid excessive fatigue. It includes adequate rest, nutrition and exercise.

     Examples: Availability of adequate rest; Maintenance of adequate nutrition.

  II. ***Conservation of structural integrity***: Refers to maintaining or restoring the structure of body preventing physical breakdown and promoting healing.

     Examples: Assist patient in ROM exercise; Maintenance of patient's personal hygiene.

  III. ***Conservation of personal integrit***y: Recognizes the individual as one who strives for recognition, respect, self-awareness, self-hood and self-determination.

     Examples: Recognize and protect patient's space needs.

  IV. ***Conservation of social integrity:*** An individual is recognized as someone who resides with in a family, a community, a religious group, an ethnic group, a political system and a nation.

     Examples: Help the individual to preserve his or her place in a family, community, and society, position patient in bed to foster social interaction with other patients, avoid sensory deprivation, promote patient's use of newspaper, magazines, radio, TV, provide support and assistance to family.

ASSUMPTIONS

Myra Levine's Model also discusses other assertions and assumptions:

- The nurse creates an environment in which healing could occur.
- A human being is more than the sum of the part.
- Human beings respond in a predictable way.
- Human beings are unique in their responses.
- Human beings know and appraise objects, condition and situation.
- Human beings sense reflects reason and understands.
- Human beings actions are self-determined even when emotional.
- Human beings are capable of prolonging reflection through such strategists raising questions.
- Human beings make decision through prioritizing course of action.
- Human being must be aware and able to contemplate objects, condition and situation.
- Human beings are agents who act deliberately to attain goal.
- Adaptive changes involve the whole individual.
- A human being has unity in his response to the environment.

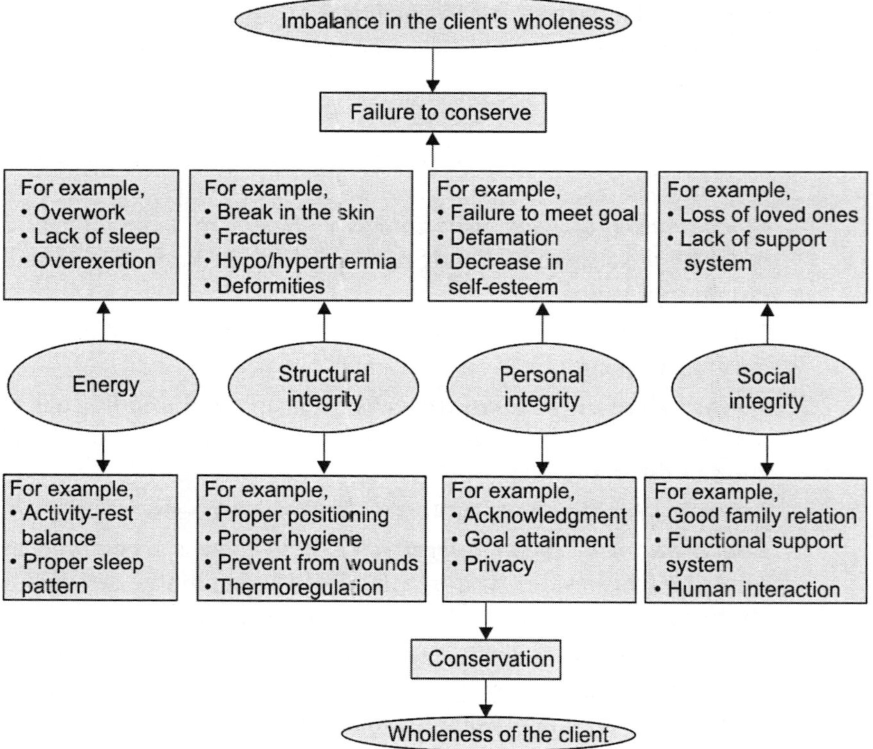

Fig. 7.1: A continuum paradigm on Myra Levine's four conservation principle

- Every person possesses a unique adaptive ability based on one's life experience which creates a unique message.
- There is an order and continuity to life change is not random.
- Human beings respond organismically in an ever changing manner.
- A theory of nursing must recognize the importance of detail of care for a single patient with in an empiric framework that successfully describe the requirement of the all patient.
- A human being is a social animal.
- A human being is a constant interaction with an ever changing society.
- Change is inevitable in life.
- Nursing needs existing and emerging demands of self-care and dependent care.
- Nursing is associated with condition of regulation of exercise or development of capabilities of providing care.

Characteristics of Theory

- The concept of illness adaptation, using interventions, and the evaluation of nursing interventions are interrelated.
- Concepts are sequential and logical and can be used to explain the consequences of nursing action.
- Levine's theory is easy to use and elements are easily comprehensible.
- Levine's idea can be tested and hypothesis can be derived from them.
- The principle of conservation are specific enough to be testable.
- Levine's idea has not yet been widely researched.
- Levine's theory has been applied in surgical settings.
- Levine's ideas are consistent with other theories, laws and principles particularly those from the humanities and sciences.

NURSING PROCESS

Assessment

- Collection of provocative facts through observation and interview of challenges to the internal and external environment using four conservation principles.
- Nurses observes patient for organismic responses to illness, reads medical reports. talks to patient and family.
- Assesses factors which challenges the individual.

Trophicognosis

- Nursing diagnosis gives provocative facts meaning.
- A nursing care judgment arrived at through the use of the scientific process.
- Judgment is made about patient's needs for assistance.

Hypothesis

- Planning
- Nurse proposes hypothesis about the problems and the solutions which becomes the plan of care.
- Goal is to maintain wholeness and promoting adaptation.

Interventions

- Testing the hypothesis
- Interventions are designed based on the conservation principles.
- Mutually acceptable.
- Goal is to maintain wholeness and promoting adaptation.

Evaluation

- Observation of **organismic response** to interventions.
- It is assesses whether hypothesis is supported or not supported.
- If not supported, plan is revised, new hypothesis is proposed.

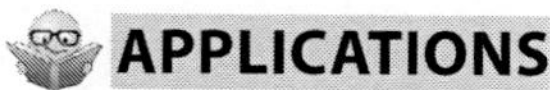

APPLICATIONS

Nursing Research

- Principles of conservation have been used for data collection in various researches.
- Conservational model was used by Hanson, et al. in their study of incidence and prevalence of pressure ulcers in hospice patient.
- Newport used principle of conservation of energy and social integrity for comparing the body temperature of infant's who had been placed on mother's chest immediately after birth with those who were placed in warmer.

Nursing Education

- Conservational model was used as guidelines for curriculum development.
- It was used to develop nursing undergraduate program at Allentown College of St Francis de Sales, Pennsylvania.
- Used in nursing education program sponsored by Kupat Holim in Israel.

Nursing Administration

- Taylor described an assessment guide for data collection of neurological patients which forms basis for development of comprehensive nursing care plan and thus evaluate nursing care.
- McCall developed an assessment tool for data collection on the basis of four conservational principles to identify nursing care needs of epileptic patients.

- Family assessment tool was designed by Lynn-McHale and Smith for families of patient in critical care setting.

Nursing Practice

- Conservational model has been used for nursing practice in different settings.
- Bayley discussed the care of a severely burned teenagers on the basis of four conservational principles and discussed patient's perceptual, operational and conceptual environment.
- Pond used conservation model for guiding the nursing care of homeless at a clinic, shelters or streets.

LIMITATION

- Limited attention is focused on health promotion and illness prevention.
- Nurse has the responsibility for determining the patient ability to participate in the care, and if the perception of nurse and patient about the patient ability to participate in care do not match, this mismatch will be an area of conflict.
- The major limitation is the focus on individual in an illness state and on the dependency of patient.
- There are a number of limitations when it comes to the four principles. On conservation of energy, Levine's goal is to avoid fatigue or excessive use of energy. This is manageable in the bedside care of ill clients. In cases where energy needs to be utilized rather than conserved like in manic patients, attention deficit hyperactivity disorder (ADHD) in children or those with limited movements such as paralyzed clients, Levine's theory does not apply.
- On conservation of structural integrity, the focus is to preserve the anatomical structure of the body as well as to prevent damage to the anatomical structure. This, again, has limitations. In cases, where the anatomical structure is not so perfect but without identified disfigurement or problems as in plastic surgeries, procedures like breast enhancements and liposuctions; the person's structural integrity is compromised but it is the patient's choice seeking physical beauty and psychological satisfaction that is taken into consideration. Otherwise such procedures should not be promoted.
- On conservation of personal integrity, the nurse is expected to provide knowledge and the patient need to be respected, provided with privacy, encouraged and psychologically supported. The limitations here will center on clients who are psychologically impaired and incapacitated and cannot comprehend and absorb knowledge, i.e. comatose patients, suicidal individuals or clients.

- Lastly, conservation of social integrity's aim is to preserve and recognition of human interaction, particularly with the clients, significant others who comprise his support system. The limitation specific for this, is when the client has no significant others like family members. Abandoned children, psychiatric patients who are unable to interact, unresponsive clients like unconscious individuals, the focus here is no longer the patient himself but the people involved in his/her health care.

CRITIQUING THE THEORY

- She values the holistic approaches to all individual, well or sick.
- Values patient's participation in nursing care.
- Comprehensive content in depth.
- Provides direction of nursing research, education, administration and practice.
- Logically congruent.
- Shows high regard to adjunctive discipline to develop theoretical basis for nursing.

USE OF THE CONSERVATION MODEL IN PRACTICE

- The model has been used to guide patient care in settings such as critical care, acute care, emergency room, primary care, long-term/extended care, homeless in the community.
- This model has been used with a variety of patients across the life-span including the neonate, infant, young child, pregnant women, young adult, long-term ventilator patient, older adult and elderly patients.
- This model has been used as a framework for wound care, managing respiratory illness, managing sleep in patient with myocardial infraction, developing nursing diagnosis and assessing for changes in bladder function.

PRACTICAL APPLICATION OF LEVINE'S MODEL

Mrs Suman, 45-year-old a wife of an abusive husband who is a coolie, underwent a radical mastectomy, postoperatively has pain, weight loss, nausea. Patient has history of smoking and stays in house which is less than sanitary. She is also depressed, has anxiety about the future and negative self-image.

Assessment

- ***Challenges to internal environment***: Weight loss, nausea.
- ***Challenges to external environment***: Abusive husband, insanitary condition in home.
- ***Energy conservation***: Weight loss, pain and nausea.

- ***Structural integrity***: Threatened by surgical procedure.
- ***Personal integrity***: Depression, anxiety and negative self-image.
- ***Social integrity***: Strained relationship with husband, financial problem.

Trophicognosis

- Inadequate nutrition
- Pain
- Potential for wound infection
- Decreased self-worth
- Potential for abuse.

Hypothesis

- Nutritional consultation
- Administration of analgesics
- Care of surgical wound
- Exploring concern regarding mastectomy.

Intervention

- ***Energy conservation***
  - Provide medication for pain and nausea.
  - Allowing rest period.
- ***Structural integrity***
  - Wound care.
  - Administrating antibiotic for wound.
- ***Personal integrity***
  - Exploring her feeling about breast removal while respecting her privacy.
- ***Social integrity***
  - Assess potential abuse from husband.
  - Support to the family.

Organismic Response

- Controlled pain
- Wound healing
- Improved appetite, weight gain
- Assistance from husband
- Decreased financial expenditure
- Improved self-image
- Decreased anxiety
- Improved knowledge.

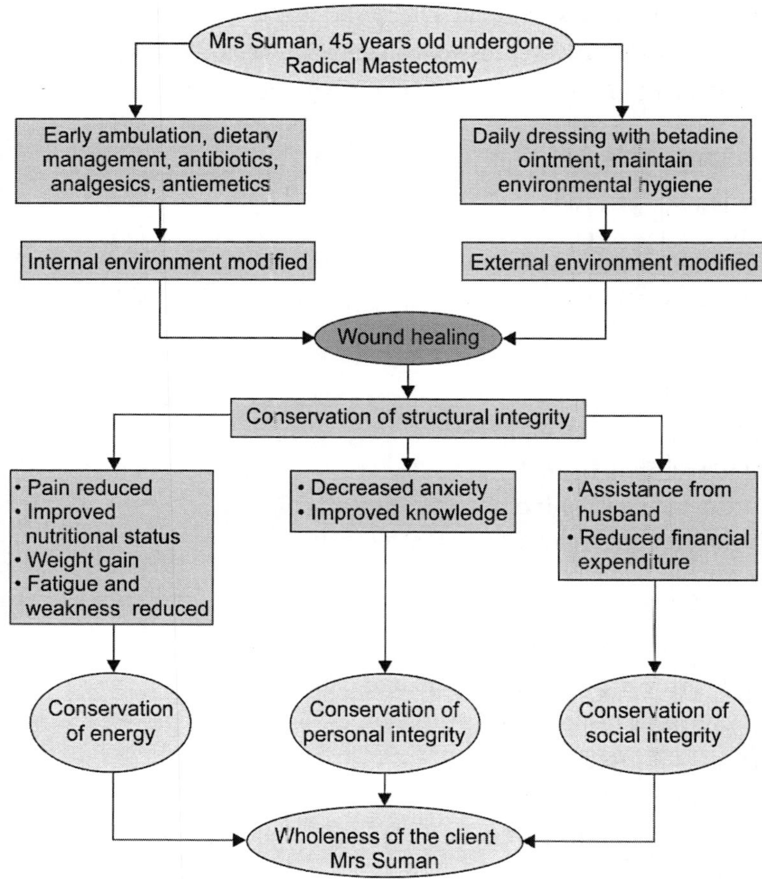

Fig. 7.2: A Continuum/paradigm on Myra Levines' four conservation principle

CONCLUSION

Levine's notion of the environment as complex provides an excellent basis for continuing to develop an improved understanding of the environment by studying the interaction between the external and internal environment, will provide for a better understanding of adaptation.

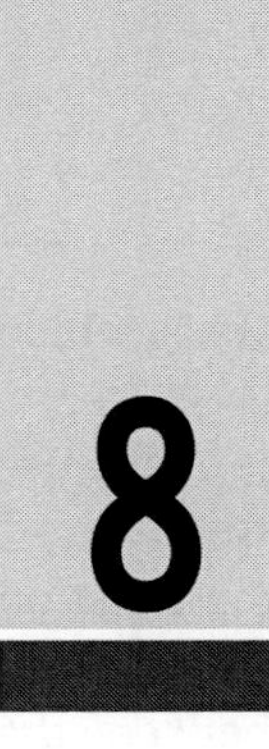

Betty Neuman: Systems Theory

INTRODUCTION

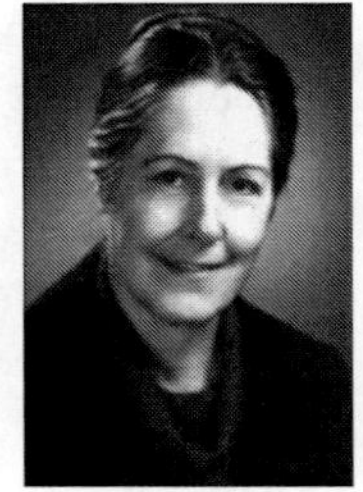

Betty Newman

Newman's model gives a framework to render nursing care in a holistic and system based manner. The primary focus is on the system's responses to the environmental stressors and use of primary, secondary, and tertiary actions in order to maintain the balance in the system.

Biography

- She was born in 1924 near Lowell, Ohio.
- She worked in different cadres of nursing in California, after receiving Registered Nurse diploma from Peoples Hospital School of Nursing, Akron, Ohio in 1947.
- In 1957, she graduated in nursing from University of California at Los Angeles along with majors in Psychology and Public health.
- She lead the way in the community health movement in the 1960s.
- Started to prepare her model while lecturer in community health nursing at University of California, Los Angeles.
- The first draft of the model was published in Nursing Research in 1972 in the name of '*A Model for Teaching Total Person Approach to Patient Problems*.' Later, she redefined it in 1972 and in 1980.
- Her model was greatly influenced by the Gestalt theory, von Bertalanffy, and Laszlo on general system theory, Selye's general adaptation Syndrome and Lazarus's stress and coping theory.
- In 1985, Pacific Western University awarded PhD in Clinical Psychology to her.
- There are various revisions of her models in the later years and the latest being done in the 2010.

Assumptions

- Human being is like an open system which is dynamic and continuous flow of energy between environment.
- Though each human system is distinctive, there are certain commonalities in certain range of responses within normal range in the basic core structure.

- Many known, unknown and universal environmental stresses exist which have the ability to disturb the system's stability.
- Stressors break the normal line of defense when the flexible line of defense fails to protect the system from the threat of environmental stressors.
- Line of resistance brings the body to normal stage after the reaction which is the aftermath of environmental stressors.
- Wellness in system is achieved through the interrelationship between the physiological, psychological, sociocultural and spiritual variables.
- *Primary prevention* aim at reducing the risk associated with environmental stressors thereby preventing the reaction. This can be achieved through early client assessment and identification.
- *Secondary prevention* focuses on sign and symptoms due to reaction and these interventions are there to mitigate the noxious effects.
- *Tertiary prevention* brings the client system into the stage of primary prevention.

Concepts

1. *Human being* is viewed as an open system that interacts with either internal and external environment forces or stressors. The human is in constant change, moving towards a dynamic state of system stability or toward illness of varying degrees.
2. *Basic structure:* This encompasses the factors that are common to the particular type of organisms. These factors include normal temperature range, genetic structure-response pattern, organ strength or weakness, ego structure.
3. *Flexible line of defense* is the protective covering which prevents the entry of stressors into the human system. Hence, it protects the normal line of defense. Factors such as multiple stressors, poor sleep pattern, poor nutrition can weaken this line.
4. *Normal line of defense* is the state of wellness. This is very essential for the nurses to determine the extent of wellness in order to rule out the level of reaction.
5. *Lines of resistance* are the series of cycles which surround the basic structure which get activated when the environmental stress crosses the normal line of defense. This line consists of known and unknown resources to fight against the stressors. For instance, factors support the body such as mobilization of white blood cells (WBCs) and activation of immune system. Those individual whose lines of resistance are weak or ineffective are prone for energy depletion and eventually to death.
6. *Stability:* It is a state of equilibrium in which the client system is able to cope with the environmental stressors thus maintains the integrity of the system.
7. *Reaction:* It is the extent of disequilibrium as the result of invasion of stressors through the normal line of defense.

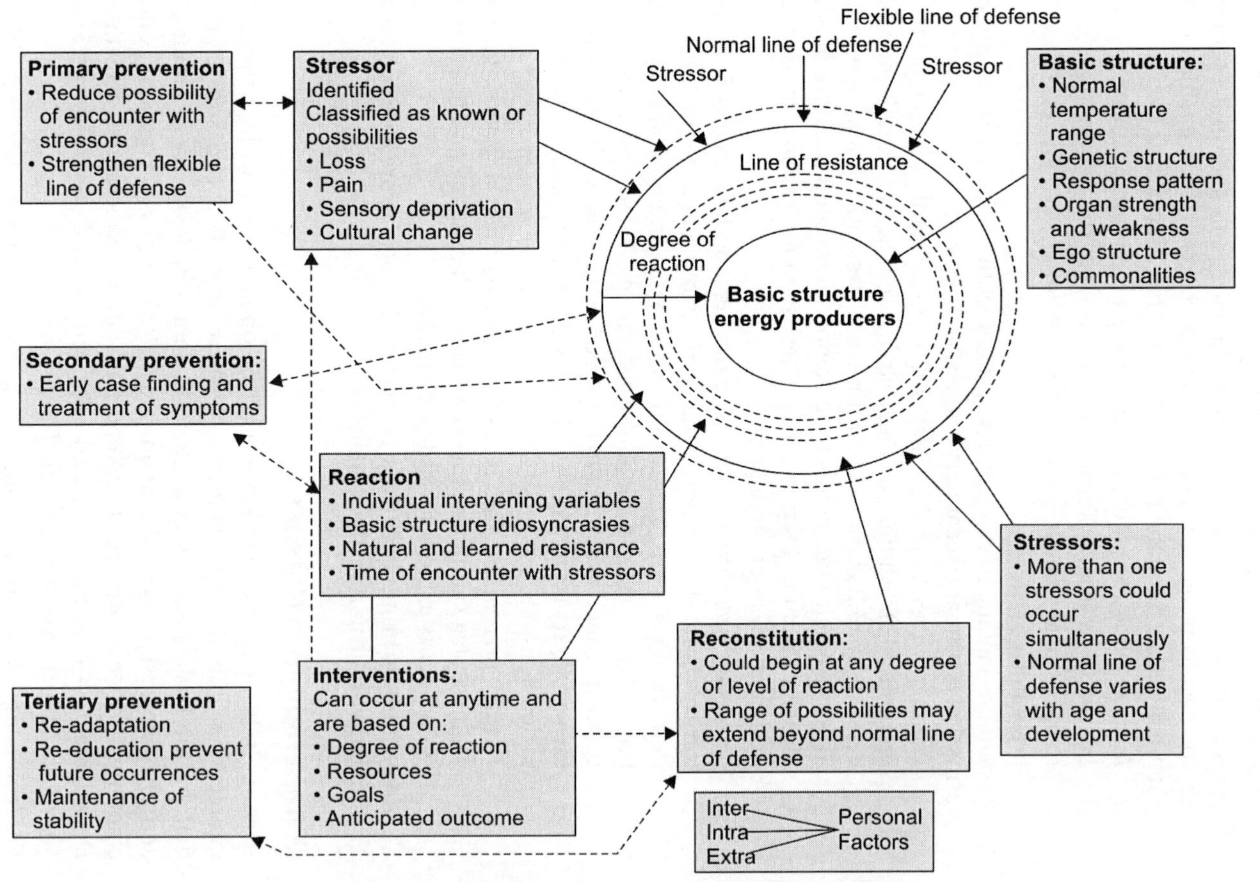

Fig. 8.1: Concepts of Betty Neuman's systems theory

8. *Entropy* is the process of energy depletion and the client system is moving toward the illness or death.
9. *Negentropy* is a balanced state of clients system which have continuous interaction of input, output and feedback.
10. *Stressors* are able to make changes in the client's system in a positive way or negative way. A stressor is any environmental force which can potentially affect the stability of the system. They may be:
    a. *Intrapersonal*—occur within person, e.g. emotions and feelings
    b. *Interpersonal*—occur between individuals, e.g. role expectations
    c. *Extrapersonal*—occur outside the individual, e.g. job or finance pressures.
11. *Prevention* encompasses the nursing interventions. It can be in three forms that is primary, secondary and tertiary prevention.
    a. *Primary prevention:* This intervention is primarily focuses on the promotion of wellness through strengthening the flexible line of defense by reduction of environmental stressors. In addition, this measure can initiate at any time before the reaction has developed. Measures such as immunization, lifestyle modifications can be the primary prevention strategies.
    b. *Secondary prevention:* Starts after the reaction has occurred in the form of sign and symptoms of the intrusion of environmental stressors into client's system. This aim to resume the internal stability and prevent the further depletion of the energy. Nursing interventions can be planned according to the need and priorities of the clients. If the secondary interventions fail to regain system stability, it can lead to death.
    c. *Tertiary prevention:* This helps the clients system to back into the wellness stage and these measures can initiate at any point after the system starts to move towards reconstitution.
12. *Reconstitution* brings back the system into the stage before illness. It also strengthens the normal line of defense.

Metaparadigm in Nursing

Person: It is in a dynamic state and an open system with reciprocal interactions with the environment. Newman identified five subsystems that are the basic elements in a clients system. *Physiological*—anatomical and physiological aspects of human body, *Psychological*— cognition, and emotions, *Sociocultural*—relationships and other sociocultural activities, *Developmental*—changes associated with growth and development and *Spiritual*—influence of spiritual beliefs.

Environment: *It* is the internal and external factors that surrounds the client system. She identifies three types of environment.

1. The *internal environment* exists within the client system.
2. The *external environment* exists outside the client system.

3. A *created environment* which is an environment that is created and developed unconsciously by the client and is symbolic of system wholeness.

***Health**: According to her, wellness and illness are on opposite side of a continuum. Those individual who achieve complete wellness is called healthy. Wellness occurs when the energy is more than its demand, while death occurs when the energy is not available to support the client system.*

Nursing: It is the fundamental responsibility of the nurses is to keep the clients system integrity. Nurses must assess the effects of stressors on system and also assess client's changes that are indispensible for the road towards wellness. Nursing actions can be done in the form of primary, secondary and tertiary interventions.

Application of The Science of Unitary Human Beings (SUBH)

Clinical Practice

- Newman's system models can be easily reproduced in all the setting and specialties.
- Nurses try the patients to reach the wellness by using various levels of interventions, whereas the clients act as participant and receiver of the nursing care.
- The system models have adopted in various hospitals and communities across the globe.

Nursing Education

It has often been selected as a curriculum guide for a conceptual framework oriented more toward wellness than toward a medical model and has been used at various levels of nursing education.

Nursing Research

This model has received global recognition as a guide for conducting various nursing activities in nursing.

Nursing Process According to Systems Theory

Neman proposed following stages in nursing process:

Nursing diagnosis: Based of necessity in a thorough assessment, and with consideration given to five variables in three stressor areas.

Nursing goals: Perceptions of both nurses and patients assessed separately and evaluated for any discrepancies.

Nursing actions: It is the primary, secondary and tertiary interventions in order to maintain the system integrity.

Nursing outcomes: Considered in relation to five variables, and achieved through primary, secondary and tertiary interventions.

Practical Application of Systems Theory

Case Scenario

Patient Profile

Mr Ravi is a 52-year-old farmer was admitted in the male medical ward with the complaints of shortness of breath since last two weeks, decreased urine output and swelling over the body since last three months.

Nursing Assessment

As perceived by Mr Ravi

- **Stressors**
  - *Major stress area or health concern:* He is suffering with breathing difficulty, swelling over the body and low urine output
  - He is diagnosed with chronic kidney disease after various diagnostic tests.
  - Patient had hospitalized with history of prostate hyperplasia and underwent surgical removal of prostate 3 years back
  - He is totally numbed about the new diagnosis and not speaking to others and wishes to be alone always.
  - He is also a know cases of hypertension since ten years and on antihypertensive drug
- **Lifestyle pattern**
  - Mr Ravi is a farmer and very keen to cultivate variety of crops in his land.
  - He is a vegetarian and love to eat homely meals always.
  - He has a supportive family and friends.
  - Smoke nicotine very occasionally, however no alcohol drinking habit.
  - Love to watch television programs and engage in various activities in his land.
  - He is an active member of local council.
- **Similar experiences in the past**
  - He told that he was very anxious and during the previous hospitalization owing to the prostate problems.
  - Support from his family and friends helped him for speedy recovery.
- **Anticipation about the future**
  - He thinks this kidney problem is a life-threatening diseases and will not be able to recover soon.
  - He also worried about the status of crops since no one is there in home to look after it
  - Anticipating about the regular follow-ups visit in future.
- **What he is doing to help himself?**
  - He said that he thinks about the best moments in his life to instill positive thoughts and avoiding negative thoughts.

- **What is expected from the others?**
  - Though he is not interacting much with family members, he wish to spend some precious time with them and his friends.
  - Expect much more cooperation and therapeutic attitude towards him from the health care professionals.
  - Have some role in participating in the therapeutic plan.

Stressors as Experiences by the Nurse

After the history collection, the assigned nurse validated the information which was given by Mr Ravi about stressors, lifestyle pattern, similar experiences, anticipation about the future, strategies adopted and expectation from the others. Nurse found that there are no any discrepancies with her assessment and patient's response.

Assessment of Client System

- *Physiological:* He is conscious and well-oriented with time, person and place. His blood pressure is 140/90 mmHg and rest of the vitals is within the normal range. His whole body is having the pitting edema most prominently on legs and upper extremities. Crackles sound is present on light lower lobe of lungs. Renal function test reveals urea: 64 mg/dL, potassium: 6.0 mEq/L, and chloride: 117 mmol/L. In addition, urine is pale yellow in color with presence of albumin. USG findings shows bilateral grade-I echogenicity in his both kidneys, urinary bladder is minimally distended and free fluid is present in peritoneal cavity.
- *Psychosocial cultural:* Mr Ravi is anxious about the progress of this life-threatening disease. He is not willing to talk about his feeling to others, however, he expects family and friends have to be with him. He is a very active member of the local council.
- *Developmental:* Patient is very much engaged in farming activities since childhood. He maintains a cordial relationship with family members
- *Spiritual:* Mr Ravi believes in Hinduism. He also trust on the existence of God and will not do anything unethical.

Nursing Diagnosis

- Ineffective breathing pattern related to diminished lung or chest expansion associated with accumulation of fluid as evidenced by altered breathing pattern.

  Nursing outcome: Patient will maintain an effective breathing pattern.

  Nursing action:

Primary prevention	Secondary prevention	Tertiary prevention
• Assess the respiratory pattern	• Evaluate the respiratory function to rule out the causes of difficulty in breathing	• Educate the patient about the importance of adherence to medication and regular follow-ups

Contd...

Contd...

Primary prevention	Secondary prevention	Tertiary prevention
• Provide a comfortable position preferably semi-Fowlers for the proper expansion of lungs • Provide a calm and restful environment • Help him to perform activities of daily living	• Assist him to make a comfortable position • Reassure him that nurses are always available to help him during any problems • Teach him about abdominal breathing or coughing exercises • Administer medication as per physician order	• Involve the patient as well as family members in treatment planning • Provide primary and secondary interventions if required

Evaluation: The goal was partially achieved as evidenced by decrease in breathing difficulty.

Critique of the Newman's Theory

Clarity: Concepts of this theory are abstract and difficult to interpret; however all the ideas are better known to the nurses.

Simplicity: Concepts of this theory are overlapping and complex in nature.

Generality: Newman's system models can be easily reproduced in all the health care setting while working for the individuals, families and communities.

Empirical precision: This model is found to be an effective guide for various researches, however, the testability of the variables of her concepts in research is still to explore.

 CONCLUSION

The Newman's system model helps the nurses to provide a comprehensive and holistic care to patients by controlling the effect of environmental stressors on the client's system. In fact, her theory has got much acceptance across the globe owing to the maintenance of client's integrity through simple three level nursing interventions.

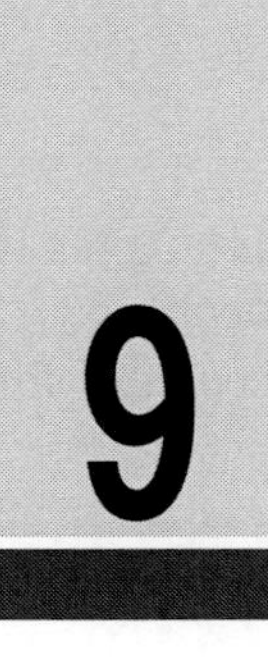

Dorothea Orem: Self-Care Deficit Theory

INTRODUCTION

It is one of the grand nursing theories which mainly focus on the self-care abilities of an individual. She identified that each individual have the ability to take care of themselves, a nurses need to assist him in maintaining health-based on his condition. This theory includes three interrelated theories, i.e. theory of self-care, self-care deficit theory and theory of nursing systems.

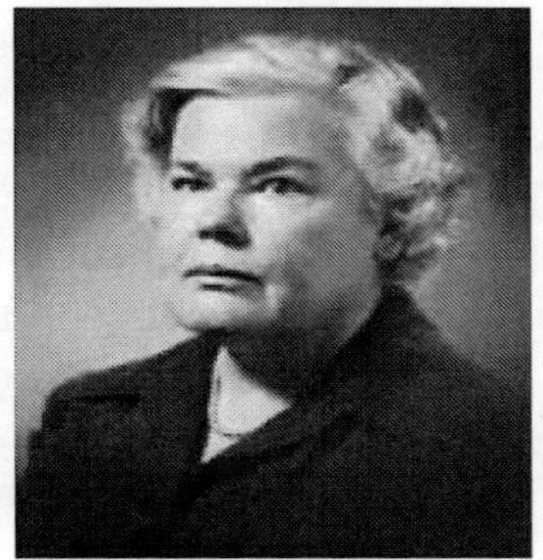

Dorothea Orem

Biography

- She was born as youngest of two daughters in Baltimore, Maryland in 1914.
- She attended a nursing diploma certificate course in 1930 from Providence School of Nursing, Washington.
- She graduated in nursing in 1939, received masters' degree in nursing from the Catholic university of America, Washington, DC.
- She worked in different caders of nursing during her career from Bedside nurse to Dean of School of Nursing and during this period, she worked on her theoretical concepts on nursing and self-care.
- She wrote a book on Nursing Practice in 1971 and has revised periodically in 1980, 1985, 1991, 1995 and 2001.
- She received PhD in Science in 1976 and 1980 from Georgetown University and Incarnate Word College, San Antonio, Texas, respectively.

Assumptions

- Human beings require continuous, deliberate inputs to themselves and their environment to remain alive and function in accordance with natural human endowments.
- Human agency has power to act deliberately in identifying needs and making inputs in the form of care for the self and others.
- People should be self-reliant and responsible for their own care and others in their family needing care.
- Mature human beings experience privations in the form of limitations for action in the care of self and others.

- Successfully meeting universal and development self-care requisites is an important component of primary care prevention and ill health.
- A person's knowledge of potential health problems is necessary for promoting self-care behaviors.

Concepts

- **Theory of self-care:** The main concepts include:

  Self-care: All the activities which is done by the individual in order to maintain health and well-being. The abilities to perform this activity are determined by age, health, resources available and various experiences in life.

  Self-care agency: It is the ones ability to perform self-care activities.

  Self-care requisites: These are the actions which is essential to maintain a balance between rest and activity. She identified in three types of self-care requisites: Universal, Developmental, and Health deviation.

  1. *Universal self-care requisites:* These are common to all the species at different stages of life. She found these eight requisites which are indispensable to maintain the structure and function of the human body.
     - The maintenance of a sufficient intake of air
     - The maintenance of a sufficient intake of water
     - The maintenance of a sufficient intake of food
     - The provision of care associated with elimination process and excrements
     - The maintenance of a balance between activity and rest
     - The maintenance of a balance between solitude and social interaction
     - The prevention of hazards to human life, human functioning, and human well-being
     - The promotion of human functioning and development within social groups in accord with human potential, known human limitations, and the human desire to be normal.
  2. *Developmental self-care requisites:* These are associated with the developmental stages of human and any new requisite that can be derived from a disease.
  3. *Health deviation self-care requisites:* These types of requisites are the result of an illness, injury and any medical procedures. A nurse must be able to identify these and able to help the patient and relatives in identifying and coping with these newly developed self-care requisites.
     - Seek out medical treatment
     - Being aware of and attending to the effects and results of pathologic conditions and states
     - Effectively carrying out medically prescribed diagnostic, therapeutic, and rehabilitative measures

- Being aware of and attending to or regulating the discomforting or deleterious effects of prescribed medical measures
- Adjusting self-concept with the disease in order to seek particular treatment
- Adapting to live with the diseases and its effects.

Therapeutic self-care demand: It is the amount of self-care actions which is to be done in order to meet the self-care requisites.

Basic conditioning factors: These are attributes that determine the self-care ability of an individual such as age, gender, health status, family, sociocultural, lifestyle, and environmental factors.

- **Theory of self-care deficit:** This theory narrates when the nursing actions are required and the way the nurses can help the patients to overcome from self-care deficit.
  - *Self-care deficit:* It is a state in which an individual is not capable of performing self-care activities or self-care demands are more than the self-care agency. Here, the nurses have to assist the individual in meeting the self-care demands.
  - *Nursing agency* is the nurses who are trained particularly for helping others in meeting self-care demands by doing various actions or developing their self-care agency.

    A nurse can help clients by the following ways:
    - Acting for or doing for another
    - Guiding and directing
    - Providing physical or psychological support
    - Providing and maintaining an environment that supports personal development
    - Teaching.

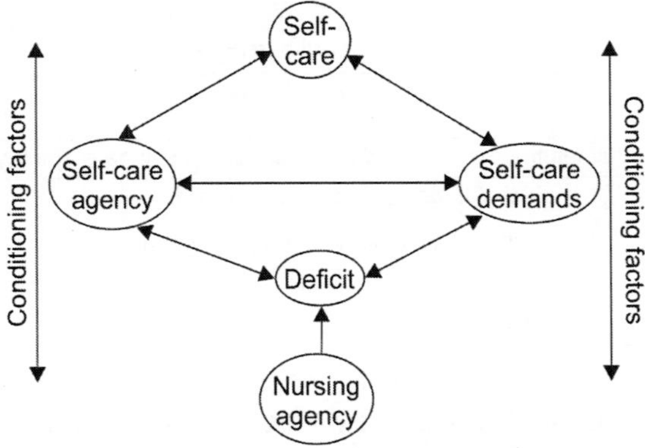

Fig. 9.1: Orem's theory of self-care deficit

- **Theory of nursing systems:** This theory explains the ways in which the patient's self-care needs are met by the nurse, patient, or both.
  - **Nursing systems:** It is a complex interaction between the nurse and patients that happen when an individual is in self-care deficit

state. She identified three levels of nursing system that is wholly compensatory, partly compensatory, and supportive-educative nursing system.

- *Wholly compensatory nursing system:* This type of nursing system is indispensible when the client is not able to do any self-care activities where nurse acts for client in performing these actions. The client may not have any active role just being the recipient of nursing care.
- *Partly compensatory nursing system:* In this, both nurse and client perform self-care actions in order to meet the self-care demands. Nurse compensates the deficiencies in the patient self-care activities.
- *Supportive-educative system:* Also called supportive-developmental system in which client is able to do self-care, however, he needs some helps of nurse in decision-making, behavior modification, and knowledge acquisition. Nurse teach the client and family about the how to promote self-care agency with the help of various tools.

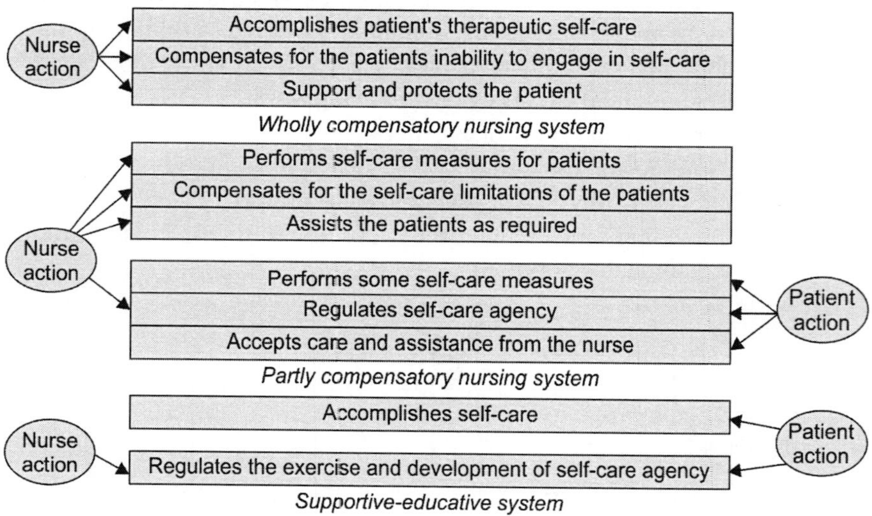

Fig. 9.2: Theory of nursing system

Metaparadigm in Nursing

Person: An individual with special needs for the maintenance of self-care thereby wellness. He is also capable for doing self-care and function biologically, symbolically and socially.

Environment: It is the surroundings of an individual which have direct effect on the self-care agency.

Health: It is the state which is structurally and functionally maintained the integrity. A healthy person or group can self-reflect, learn from experience and socialize with others.

Nursing: This is the specialized actions by trained nurses to help clients in doing self-care activities in order to maintain the integrity. Nurse identify the self-care deficit of clients and plan nursing interventions accordingly.

Application of Orem's Theory

- *Nursing practice:* This theory is applied in nursing for finding the relationship between the self-care agency and nursing agency. Furthermore, this framework gives guidelines to plan various nursing activities based on patient's self-care deficit. The main areas of nursing activities include:
  - Maintaining nurse-patient relationship
  - Determining how patient can be helped through nursing
  - Responding to patient requests, desires and needs
  - Providing and regulating direct help to patient
  - Coordinating and integrating nursing with patients daily living
- *Nursing education:* Orem's theory has been implemented in many nursing curriculum. It helps the nurses to implement nursing actions in nursing process, and various methods to evaluate the effectiveness of nursing curriculum.
- *Nursing research:* Has used in various researches in order to test the efficacy of nursing agency on patients outcomes.

Nursing process according to Orem's Theory

Step 1 : *Assessment:* Complete assessment of patient health status, self-care ability and requirements along with patient's and doctor's perspectives.

Step 2 : *Nursing diagnosis and planning:* Nurses proposes a system which is based on the patient's self-care ability and select various methods of helping patients to overcome his self-care deficit.

Step 3 : *Implementation and evaluation:* Nurse helps the clients or family to accomplish integrity based on his needs. Later, she also evaluates the outcome of nursing actions.

Case scenario

Mrs Rani is admitted in the surgical ward with complaint of left side neck swelling, unexplained diarrhea. These problems have tormented her since three months. After the initial examination and investigation, physician prescribed for biopsy and confirmed the diagnosis of papillary carcinoma thyroid. She had undergone total thyroidectomy four days before.

Step 1: Assessment

- Basic conditioning factors:
  - *Age:* 32 years
  - *Gender:* Female

- *Health state:* Health deviation due to carcinoma
- *Health care system:* Primary Health Center and District Hospital
- *Family:* Married, Supportive
- *Pattern of living:* Homemaker
- *Environment:* Remote areas with no proper sanitary facilities
- *Resources:* Family support, basic health facilities are easily accessible

- Universal self-care requisites:
  - *Air:* Breaths normally, however slight pain during breathing due to stretching at the operation site and risk for suffocation related to bleeding or edema.
  - *Water:* Poor intake of water owing to the additional intravenous (IV) fluid
  - *Food:* Vegetarian, weight 50 kg which is adequate
  - *Elimination:* Normal elimination
  - *Activity:* Pain at the surgical incision, low activities of daily living (ADL) due to hospitalization
  - *Social Interaction:* Maintain a cordial relationship with family members as well as neighbors
  - *Prevention:* Knowledge deficit in diet, ADL and sanitation.
- Developmental self-care requisites:
  - Able to manage developmental tasks of each period
  - Need assistance in ADL due to disease condition.
- Health deviation self-care requisites:
  - Poor knowledge regarding the disease and its complications
  - Adherence to the therapeutic regimen
  - Worried about postsurgical recovery
  - Adjusted with the limited movements of the body due to surgery.

Step 2: Nursing Diagnosis and Planning

Step 3: Implementation and Evaluation

Nursing diagnosis	Outcome	Nursing system	Implementation	Evaluation
Risk for suffocation related to hemor-rhage, edema	She will maintain a less risk of getting airway ob-struction	Partly com-pensatory	• Monitor the respiratory functions and surgical site • Caution her about to avoid bending neck • Provide pillow to sup-port neck • Assist in repositioning and deep breathing exercise • Perform suctioning if prescribed • Humidify the room air	Ms Rani breaths normally

Critique of Orem's Theory

Clarity: Though, her theory is based on the concept self-care, certain terms in this has created difficulty to understand due to overlapping different terms having almost same meaning.

Simplicity: It is very simple when patient is not able to care for himself, nurse will take care those task. However, the detailed analysis can show how complex it is to be one of the popular grand theories.

Generality: Despite grand theories are very difficult to implement in practice, Orem's theory has implemented successfully in many settings. The rationales behind many nursing practices are the concepts of her theory.

Empirical Precision: Orem believed that testing of her theory is not essential to prove the efficacy. But, many researchers have used it in various researches and found suitable for testing effect of nursing practice.

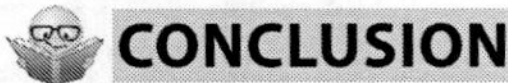

CONCLUSION

Orem's theory focuses on patient's ability to perform self-care for maintaining the integrity. Nurse assesses the patient's this ability and plan interventions accordingly.

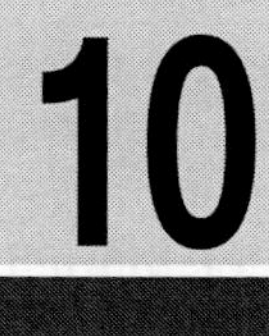

Martha Rogers: The Science of Unitary Human Beings

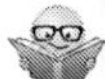

INTRODUCTION

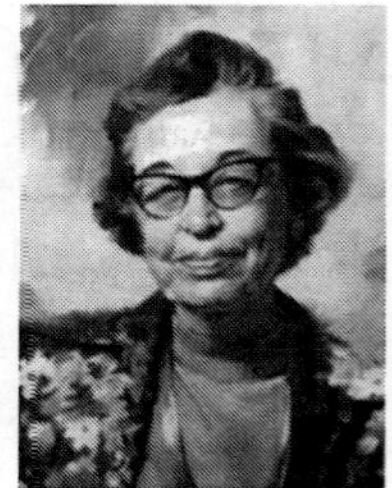
Martha Rogers

Martha Roger's theory 'The Science of Unitary Human Beings (SUBH)' is mainly focusing on the four concepts and three principles of homeodynamics that are energy fields, openness, pattern, pandimensional, integrality, resonancy, and helicy respectively. Her theory was very controversial, not been proven on scientific basis and often been accused of pseudoscience.

Biography

- She was born in Dallas, Texas, May 12, 1914; sharing her birthday with Florence Nightingale.
- Her family moved to Knoxville, Tennessee before she turned one.
- As a young child, she was very inquisitive to gain more and more knowledge, she had passion of reading books.
- In 1936, she attended nursing diploma program at Knoxville General Hospital.
- She continued her schooling at George Peabody College and completed Bachelors of Science in Public Health Nursing in 1937.
- She worked as a Public Health Nurse for two years after obtaining degree in Public Health Nursing.
- After completing her Master's in Public Health Nursing from Teachers College, Columbia University in 1946, she started working as a Public Health Nurse.
- She worked as director of Visiting Nurses Association in Phoenix, Arizona.
- In 1951, she joined Johns Hopkins University, Baltimore and completed Doctor of Science in 1954 while she was working at Catholic University.
- After completing her Doctor of Science, she served as the Head of the Division of nursing at New York University.
- In 1963, she edited the second journal in Nursing i.e. *Nursing Science.*
- *An Introduction to the Theoretical Basis of Nursing* was the most famous work of Rogers which was published in 1970. It was mainly focusing on the human interaction and nursing process.
- In 1975, she retired as Head of the Division of nursing from New York University.

- She joined Emeritus University in 1979 as a Professor and continued to work on The Science of Unitary Human Beings till the time of her demise in March 13, 1994.

THE SCIENCE OF UNITARY HUMAN BEINGS (SUBH)

Rogers does not have a specific theory on nursing, in fact what she made an abstract system specific to nursing from which many theories are derived. Rogers considered nursing as an art and science. The science of nursing is the body of knowledge emerging from scientific research and analysis. This theory provides a new frame for the nursing in education, practice and research.

Assumptions

- Human being is considered as whole which cannot be viewed as subparts.
- The life process of human is irreparable and one way, i.e. from birth to death.
- Health and illness are the continuous expression of the life process.
- The energy flows freely between the individual and environment.
- Human being possesses the ability to think, imagine, sense, feel, and can use language for expression.
- Human beings have the ability to adapt according to the new changes in the environment.

Concepts

There are four main concepts of SUBH named energy fields, openness, pattern, and pandimensional. All the human beings are viewed as an integral part of universe. Human beings and the environment have energy field, nursing action is directed towards patterning and maintaining these energy fields.

- *Energy fields:* It is the inevitable part of life. Human and environment both have energy field which is open i.e. energy can freely flow between human and environment.
- *Openness:* There is no boundary or barrier that can inhibit the flow of energy between human and environment which leads to the continuous movement or matter of energy.
- *Pattern:* It is the distinguishing character of the energy field.
- *Pandimensional:* Undeviating field which is not constricted by space or time, it is an infinite domain without boundary.

Principles of Homeodynamics

Homeodynamics refers to the balance between the dynamic life process and environment. These principles help to view human as unitary human being. The three separate principles are integrality, resonancy, and helicy.

Principle of integrality: Energy fields are dynamic and constantly interact with the human and environment, which affects our environment and vice versa. This is the principle on which meditation and humor works to produce a positive environment.

Principle of resonancy: Constant change in the way or pattern of the energy field from a lower to higher frequency. This movement of energy can be made by human touch, guided imagery activities, drawing, storytelling and other active use of imagination.

Principle of helicy: Any minute change in the environment which leads to ripple effect i.e. results in a larger changes in other field. This change is constant, unpredictable and there are many factors which mutually interact and cause the change.

Metaparadigm in Nursing

Person: A unitary human being is open systems which continuously interact with environment. A person cannot be viewed as parts, it should be considered as a whole.

Environment: It includes the entire energy field other than a person. These energy fields are irreducible, not limited by space and time, identified by its pattern and organization.

Health: Not clearly defined by Roger. It is determined by the interaction between energy fields, i.e. human and environment. Bad interaction or misplacing of the energy leads to illness.

Nursing: It is both science and art. It constantly maintains the energy field which is conducive for patient. Nursing action directs the interaction of person and environment to maximize health potential.

Application of SUBH

Clinical Practice

- Nursing is a profession, art and science.
- Nursing action is always focused on unitary human being and change the energy field between human and environment.

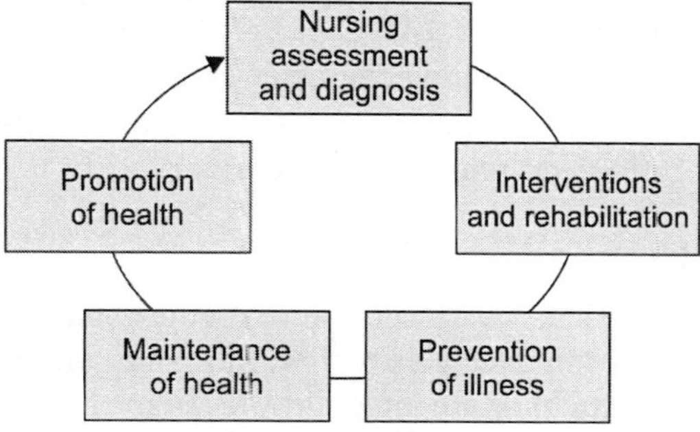

Fig. 10.1: Nursing action as per SUBH

- Nursing interventions include all the noninvasive actions such as guided imaginary, humor, therapeutic touch, music, etc. which are used to increase the potential of human being.
- The more importance should be on the management of pain, supportive psychotherapy and rehabilitation of the human being.
- Better understanding of the human is more important than giving isolated interventions. People are made aware about their thinking, emotions, and patterning of their energy field.

Nursing Research

- According to Rogers, basic research brings new knowledge, whereas applied research tests the knowledge which is already available.
- Rogerian theory has been used in many research works and has always been found testable and applicable in research.

Nursing Education

- Training in nursing should be professional and technical; emphasis should be given on the understanding of the patient and self, energy field and environment.
- Training should lay more focus on teaching non-invasive modalities such as therapeutic touch, meditation, humor, regular in-service education program, etc.

Nursing Administration

- Nurses and nursing care are playing a pivotal role in health care delivery system to promote and maintain the health of human being.
- A nurse administrative should be highly qualified in nursing, willing to bring innovative changes and have a sound knowledge in research.
- Administrators should create a conducive environment for working which will enhance the care provided by the staff members and ultimately clients well-being.

Nursing Process According to SUBH

Assessment

- Assess the general condition of the clients and environment including the changes in the life process.
- Supportive data can be collected through results of laboratory tests and disease pathology.

Pattern Appraisal

- It is an inclusive assessment of human and environment energy fields, its organization of energy field, and identification of areas of dissonance.
- Insightful reflection of nursing action.
- Nurses validate the entire appraisal along with the client.

Mutual Patterning

- It is the proper patterning of the energy fields between the human and environment.
- It is the mutual interaction between the client and nurse.
- Patterning can be done by suggesting the various alternatives, educating, empowering, encouraging, etc. depending on the client's condition and needs.
- Pattern appraisal include appraisal of nutrition, rest and sleep, exercises, discomfort, and relation with others.
- The pattering activities can be therapeutic touch, meditation, humor, imaginary, etc.

Evaluation

- Evaluation is done by repeating the pattern appraisal after the mutual patterning to determine the extents of dissonance and harmony.

PRACTICAL APPLICATION OF SUBH MODEL

Clinical scenario: Mr X is a 54-year-old male admitted in the male psychiatric ward with the diagnosis of major depression secondary to the diagnosis of Myocardial Infraction (MI). He was very tense and sobbing during the history collection. He was accompanied by his wife and son. Even though his wife was anxious but still she was supportive and helpful. Mr X was diagnosed with MI four months back and underwent the angioplasty three months ago. Currently, he was on Statins and Antihypertensives. He started to show the sing and symptoms of depression from the past one month. He used to sit alone, diminished the activities of daily living, regular crying spells, decreased chat, self-muttering, insomnia, anorexia, body aches, least bothered about personal hygiene, two days before he attempted suicide by hanging on ceiling fan. His present findings based on the assessment shows that he is very tearful, socially withdrawn, nutritional status is impaired, crying spells, sad mood, and risk for committing suicide.

Nursing Process for Mr X Based on SUBH Model (Fig. 10.2)

Critique of the SUBH

Critiquing of SUBH can be done by analyzing the five main components, i.e *simplicity, clarity, generality, and empirical precision of a theory.*

Simplicity: Although the concepts seems to quite difficult to understand. It is a parsimonious theory. Parsimony refers to theory based on simple assumption but proves to be very valuable.

Clarity: Overall Rogerian SUBH is considered as complex but still efforts are going on to clarify the complex concepts.

Assessment (pattern appraisal)	Mutual patterning	Evaluation
Mr X is experiencing the pattern of dissonance, i.e. depression with suicidal ideation, MI, pain, fear, sleep pattern disturbances, impaired nutritional status, tendencies to commit suicide and appraisal is essential for all of these symptoms.	• It is the mutual interaction between Mr X and nurse for changing the pattern and making his all emerging pattern as unitary pattern. • Therapeutic touches, meditation, guided imagery, are the pattering activities planned for Mr X. • Therapeutic touch is implemented which will cure the pain, promote the speedy recovery and building trust on nurse. • Social withdrawn can be managed by using humor, participating in small group activities and this will help him to develop self-confidence. • Advices are given for changing the dietary pattern and improving the personal hygiene. • Involvement of family for the environment pattering.	• Repeating the pattern appraisal after the mutual patterning to determine the extents of dissonance and harmony. • Current symptoms experiencing by Mr X is shared with him and if changes is needed in the mutual patterning that can be incorporated or implement the same.

Fig. 10.2: Nursing process of Mr X as per SUBH

Generality: The uses on non-invasive modalities are very useful and important to nursing even today. SUBH is the foundation of many theories and it can be apply in a variety of setting and all spheres of life.

Empirical precision: Rogerian theory has been used in many research works and has been found testable and applicable in research. But, many limitations have also been identified by the researchers such as difficult to understand the concepts, lack of operational definitions and instruments for the proper evaluation of the instruments.

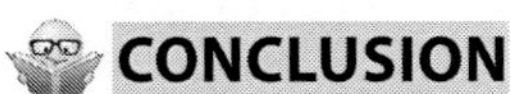

CONCLUSION

SUBH leads to a new way of seeing the person as a unitary human being and new style of nursing practice. This model is applicable in all the setting and every spheres of life. Rogers emphasized the need for noninvasive nursing modalities in achieving the health potential, it is very evident in today's situation that there is more focus on the alternative system of medicine and noninvasive nursing actions are in getting much importance.

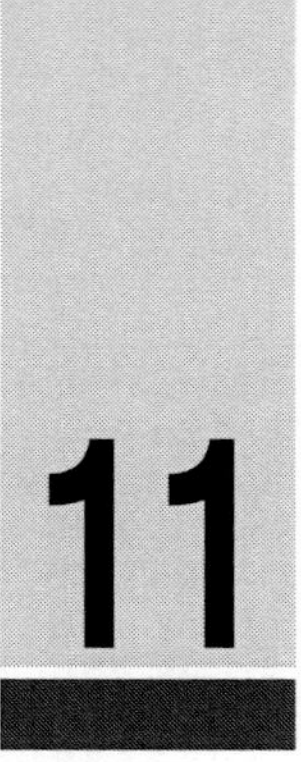

11 Callista Roy: Adaptation Theory

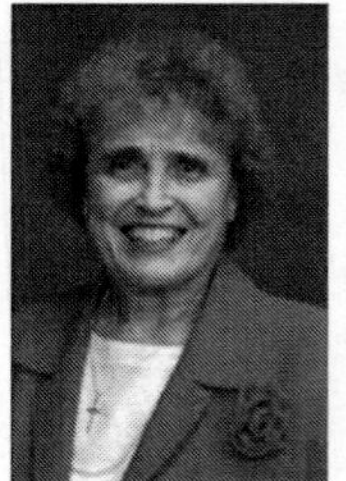

'When push comes to a shove, we will seldom disappoint ourselves. We all harbor greater stores of strength than we think. Adversity brings the opportunity to test our mettle and discover for ourselves the stuff of which we are made.'

–Callista Roy

INTRODUCTION

Sister Callista Roy developed the Adaptation Model, a prominent grand nursing theory in 1976. In Roy's model the human being has a set of interrelated systems (biological, psychological and social) and strives to maintain a balance between these systems and the outside environment, but there is no absolute level of balance. Human being strives to live within a unique group in which he or she can cope adequately.

Biography and Achievements

- Sister Callista Roy born on October 14, 1939 at Los Angeles, California.
- She started working at the age of 14 in a large hospital.
- She completed Bachelor of Arts with a major in nursing in 1963 from Mount Saint Mary's College, Los Angeles.
- She received Master's Science in pediatric nursing from University of California, Los Angeles in 1966.
- She earned her MA and PhD in Sociology in 1973 and 1977 respectively from University of California.
- Postdoctoral Fellow–University of California in San Francisco (1983—1985).
- She is a nurse theorist, writer, lecturer, researcher and teacher.
- She was Professor and Nurse Theorist at the Boston College of Nursing in Chestnut Hill.
- She had worked with Dorothy E. Johnson who helped her to develop this adaptation model while pursuing her Master's Degree.
- She also worked as faculty of Mount Saint Mary's College in 1966.
- She had organized course content according to a view of person and family as adaptive systems.
- Roy's adaptation model (RAM) as a basis of curriculum at Mount Saint Mary's College and model was implemented in Mount Saint Mary's School in 1970.

- She was made Chair of the Nursing Department at the College in 1971.
- She was a member of the Sisters of Saint Joseph of Carondelet.
- At present, she is a professor at William F. Connell School of Nursing at Boston College; she teaches at both undergraduate and graduate levels.
- Many books and articles published by her.
- She has many Honorary Doctorate Degrees and awards in excellence in fostering professional nursing standards.
- Sister Callista Roy has also been recognized as a living legend.

Assumptions

- **Scientific Assumptions:**
  - Systems of matter and energy progress to higher levels of complex self-organization.
  - Consciousness and meaning are constructive of individual and environment integration.
  - Awareness of self and environment is rooted in thinking and feeling.
  - Human beings decisions are accountable for the integration of creative processes.
  - Thinking and feeling mediate human action.
  - System relationships include acceptance, protection, and fostering of interdependence.
  - Individual and the earth have common patterns and integral relationships.
  - Individual and environment transformations are created in human consciousness.
  - Integration of human being and environment meanings results in adaptation.
- **Philosophical Assumptions:**
  - Individual has mutual relationships with the world and God.
  - Human being meaning is rooted in the omega point convergence of the universe.
  - God is intimately revealed in the diversity of creation and is the common destiny of creation.
  - Individual use human creative abilities of awareness, enlightenment, and faith.
  - Individual are accountable for the processes of deriving, sustaining, and transforming the universe.
- **Cultural Assumptions:**
  - Experience within a specific culture will influence how each element of the Roy Adaptation Model is expressed.
  - Within a culture, there is a concept that is central to the culture and that will influence some or all of the elements of the Roy Adaptation Model to a less or greater extent.

- Cultural expressions of the elements of the Roy Adaptation Model may lead to changes in practice activities likes nursing assessment.
- As Roy Adaptation Model elements evolve within a cultural perspective, implications or education and research may differ from the experience in the original culture.

METAPARADIGM

Person

- According to Callista Roy, 'Human systems have thinking and feeling capacities, rooted in consciousness and meaning, by which they adjust effectively to changes in the environment and, in turn, affect the environment.'
- Humans beings are holistic that are in constant interaction with their environment.
- Human being use a system of adaptation, both innate and acquired, to respond to the environmental stimuli they experience.
- Human systems may be individuals or groups, likes families, organizations, and the whole global community.
- Human being is the recipient of nursing care.

Environment

- According to her, environment means 'The conditions, circumstances and influences surrounding and affecting the development and behavior of persons or groups, with particular consideration of the mutuality of person and health resources that includes focal, contextual and residual stimuli.'
- Contextual stimuli are characterized as the rest of the stimuli that present with the focal stimuli, and contribute to its effect. Residual stimuli are the additional environmental factors present within the situation, but its effect is unclear (previous experience with certain stimuli).

Health

- Roy describes, 'Health is not freedom from the inevitability of death, disease, unhappiness, and stress, but the ability to cope with them in a competent way.'
- Health is defined as the state where human beings can continually adapt to stimuli. Because illness is a part of life, health is the result of a process where health and illness can coexist. If human being can continue to adapt holistically, they will be able to maintain health to reach completeness and unity. If persons cannot adapt hence, the integrity of the person can be affected negatively.
- Health is the result of process and human beings are striving to attain their maximum potential.

Nursing

- 'The goal of nursing' is the promotion of adaptation for human beings and groups in each of the four adaptive modes (physiological, self-concept, role function, and interdependence), thus contributing to health, quality of life, and dying with dignity.
- Nurses act as facilitators of adaptation. They assess the client's behaviors for adaptation; promote positive adaptation by enhancing environment interactions and helping clients react positively to stimuli. Nurses eliminate ineffective coping mechanisms and eventually lead to better outcomes for the clients.

Major Concepts of Roy's Adaptation Model

- *System:* According to Roy system is defined as a set of parts so related or connected as to form a unity or whole and also system characterized by inputs, outputs, and control and feedback processes.
- *Adaptation:* Adaptation is the 'process and outcome whereby thinking and feeling persons as individuals or in groups use conscious awareness and choice to create human and environmental integration.'
- *Adaptation level:* Adaptation level of an individual means a constantly changing point, made up of *focal, contextual, and residual stimuli,* which represent the individual's own condition of life processes.
- *Adaptation problems:* According to Roy Adaptation problem means the occurrence of a state due to inadequate responses to need deficit or excesses.
- *Stimuli:*
  - *Focal stimuli:* Focal stimuli means which immediately confront the individual.
  - *Contextual stimuli:* Contextual stimuli means which are all other stimuli present that contribute to the effect of the focal stimuli.
  - *Residual stimuli:* Residual stimuli mean environmental factors within or without the human system. These factors have effect on behavior but are effect is not validated.
- *Levels of Adaptation:*
  - *Integrated process:* The modes and subsystems meet the needs of the environment which include stable processes (e.g. spiritual realization, breathing, successful relationship).
  - *Compensatory process:* The cognator and regulator are challenged by the needs of the environment, but trying to meet the needs (e.g. starting with a new job, grief, compensatory breathing).
  - *Compromised process:* The various modes and subsystems are not sufficiently meeting the environmental challenge (e.g. unresolved loss, hypoxia, abusive relationships).
- *Internal processes (subsystem):*
  - *Regulator:* The regulator subsystem means physiological coping mechanism of an individual. It means the attempt of the body to

adapt by means of regulation of bodily processes of neurochemical and endocrine systems.

- *Cognator:* The cognator subsystem means mental coping mechanism of an individual. An individual uses his/her brain to cope by means of self-concept, interdependence, and role function adaptive modes.

- *Coping Process*
  - *Innate coping mechanism:* Means genetically determined or inherited to the species and viewed as automatic processes (inborn).
  - *Acquired coping mechanisms:* Means developed throughout strategies such as learning (acquired through life experiences).
- *Four adaptive (effector) modes:* The adaptive modes of the subsystem mean how the regulator and cognator mechanisms are manifested, i.e. they are the external expressions of the regulator and cognator and internal processes.
  - *Physiological-physical mode:* It means behavior pertaining to the physical aspect of the human system. Physical and chemical processes involved in the function and behavior of living organisms. These are the actual processes put in action by the regulator subsystem. The basic need of this mode is consist of the needs associated with oxygenation, nutrition, elimination, activity and rest, and protection. The complexes processes of this mode are linked with the, fluid and electrolytes, neurologic function, endocrine function and senses.
  - *Self-concept-group identity mode:* In this mode, sense of unity is the goal of coping, which means the purposefulness in the universe, as well as a sense of identity integrity. This consist of physical self (body image and self-ideals) and personal self (self-consistency, self-ideal, moral and ethical self).
  - *Role function or performance mode:* This mode focuses on the primary, secondary and tertiary roles of an individual that occupies in society, and understands where the individual stands as a member of society. Behaviors in this mode are described as instrumental or expressive. Instrumental behaviors are usually physical, have a long-term orientation, and focus on role mastery. Expressive behavior represents the feelings or attitude are usually emotional, and seek immediate response.
  - *Interdependence Mode:* This mode includes behavior pertaining to interdependent relationships of individuals and groups. It is mainly focus on the close relationships of people and their purpose. It involves the willingness and ability to give to others and also accept from others like love, respect and value. This is attained through effective communication and relations.
- *Adaptive responses:* Responses that promotes integrity in terms of the goals of the human system.
- *Ineffective responses:* Responses that do not contribute to integrity in terms of the goals of the human system.

- *Integrated life process:* It means structures and functions of a life process are working as a whole to meet human needs.
- *Perception:* It means the interpretation of a stimulus and the conscious appreciation of it.

THEORETICAL ASSERTIONS

The adaptive system of an individual has ***input*** (stimuli and adaptation level), **control *process*** (coping mechanism, subsystem: regulator and cognator) ***effectors*** (four adaptive mode) and ***output*** as behavioral response (may be adaptive or ineffective responses) that serve as feedback.

- *Input:* Input of the system include the three types of stimuli (focal, contextual, and residual stimuli) and adaptation level of the person. The adaptive system has input is from external environment or from the individual itself. At particular point in time these three stimuli combine and interface to set the adaptation level of the individual. This response is unique to each individual and adaptation level of each individual is regularly changing.

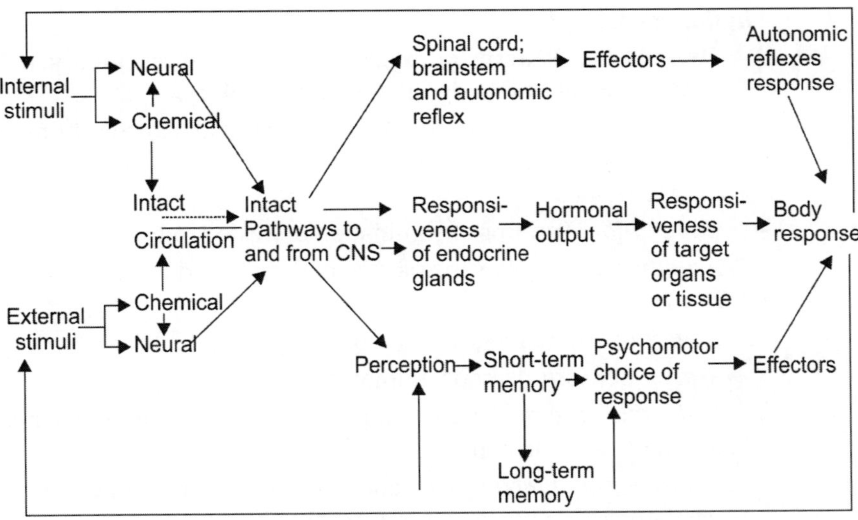

Fig. 11.1: Roys adaptation model

- *Output:* Output of the system means behavior response of the individual and that serve as feedback. It can be both internal and external. Behavior response may be adaptive response or ineffective response.
- *Control process:* It includes coping mechanism and internal process or subsystem (regulator and cognator). Coping mechanism may be innate (inherited) or acquired (learning). Regulator coping process is involving neural, chemical, and endocrine and cognator coping process is involving four cognitive emotive channel; perceptual and information processing, learning, judgment and emotion.

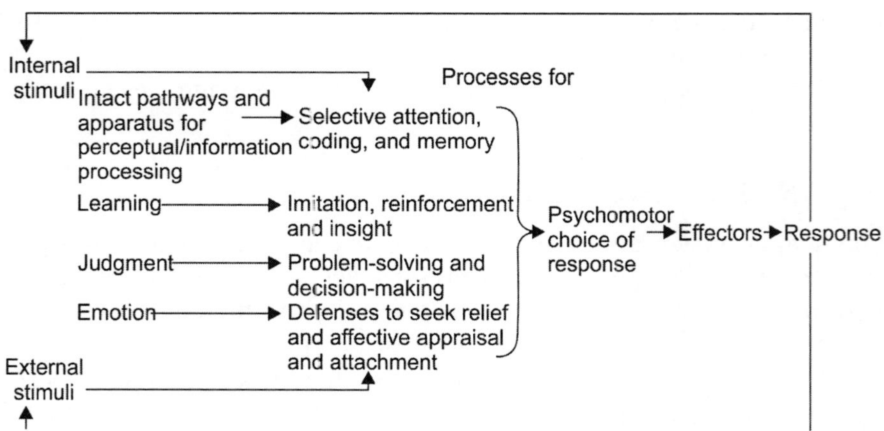

Fig. 11.2: Roys adaptation model (First figure is detailed one)

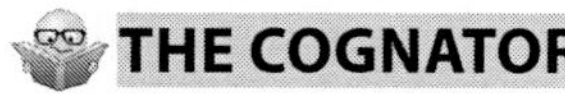

THE COGNATOR

- **Effectors**:
  - ***Physiological mode:***
    - *Oxygenation:* Patterns of oxygen use related to respiratory and cardiovascular physiology and pathophysiology.
    - *Nutrition:* Patterns of nutrient used to maintain effective human functioning and how the nutrient help for growth and repairing injured tissue.
    - *Elimination:* Patterns of elimination of waste products.
    - *Activity and rest:* How the pattern of activity and rest takes place in an individual.
    - *Protection:* Skin integrity and immunity.
    - *Senses:* Sensory-perceptual information.
    - *Fluid and electrolyte:* How the fluid and electrolyte balance maintained in the body
    - *Neurological function:* Relationship of neural function to regulator and cognator coping mechanism.
    - *Endocrine function:* How the endocrine system act in conjunction with nervous system to maintain control of the body process.
  - ***Self-concept mode:*** Which include *physical Self* (involves body sensation and body image) and *Personal Self* (made up of self-consistency, self- ideal or expectancy and the moral-ethical-spiritual self)
    - *Body sensation:* How the individual experiences the physical self.
    - *Body image:* How the individual views the physical self.
    - *Self-consistency:* Individual's efforts to maintain self-organization and to avoid disequilibrium.

  - *Self-ideal or expectancy:* Represents what the individual expects to be and do.
  - *Moral-ethical-spiritual self:* Represents individual's belief system and self-evaluation.
- ***Role function mode:***
  - *Primary role:* Which determines the majority of individual's behaviors and is defined by the individual's sex, age, and developmental stages?
  - *Secondary role:* Carry out the tasks required by the stages of development and primary role.
  - *Tertiary role:* These roles are temporary, feely chosen, and may include activities related to hobbies.
- ***Interdependence mode:*** It draws specific relationships. The first is with significant others, individual who are the most important to the him/her. The second is with support systems that is contributing to meeting interdependence needs.

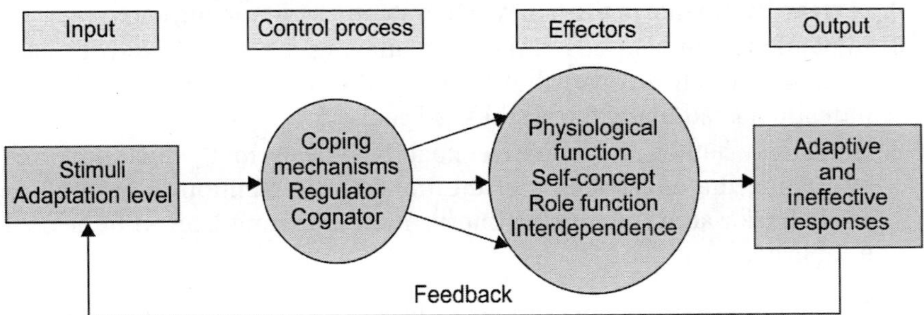

Fig. 11.3: Person as an adaptive system

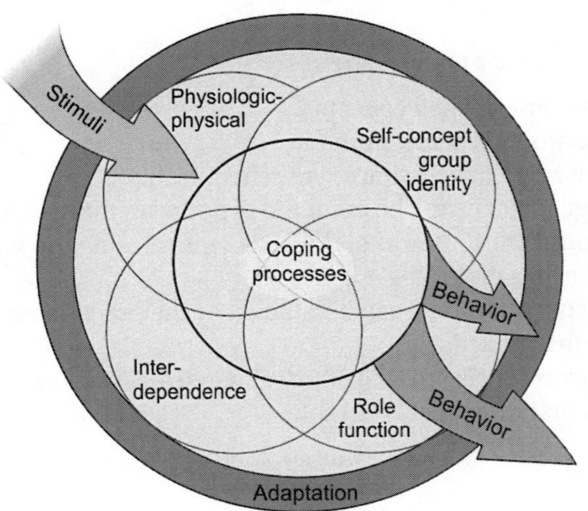

Fig. 11.4: Human adaptive system

 SIX-STEP NURSING PROCESS

A nurse's role in the Adaptation Model is to manipulate stimuli by removing, decreasing, increasing or altering stimuli so that the patient:

1. Assess the behaviors manifested from the four adaptive modes (first level assessment) which involve gathering data about the behavior of the individual as an adaptive system in each of the adaptive modes.
2. Assess the stimuli; categorize them as focal, contextual, or residual (second level assessment) which involves the identification of internal and external stimuli that are influencing the individual's adaptive behaviors.
3. Make a statement or nursing diagnosis of the individual's adaptive state which involves the formulation of statements that interpret data about the adaptation status of the individual, including the behavior and most relevant stimuli.
4. Set a goal to promote client's adaptation which involves the establishment of clear statements of the behavioral outcomes for nursing care.
5. Implement interventions aimed at managing the stimuli and to meet the goals which involves the determination of how best to assist the individual in attaining the established goals.
6. Evaluate whether the adaptive goal has been met which involves evaluating the effectiveness of the nursing intervention in relation to the behavior after the nursing intervention in comparison with the goal established.

Throughout the nursing process, based on the patient's progress toward health, the nurse and other health care professionals should make adaptations to the nursing care plan.

Characteristics of the Theory

- Theory has interrelated concepts.
- This theory is logical in nature.
- This theory is relatively simple yet generalizable.
- Roy's theory can be the basis for the hypotheses that can be tested.
- This theory contributes to and assists in increasing the general body of knowledge of a discipline.
- Roy's adaptation model can be utilized by the practitioners to guide and improve their practice.
- This theory is consistent with other validated theories, laws and principles.
- Roy's adaptation model is testable.

Application

Nursing Practice

- The Roy adaptation model is one of most frequently used conceptual frameworks used to guide nursing practice.

- With use of Roy's six step nursing process, the nurse can perform the following six functions:
  a. Assesses the behaviors manifested from the four adaptive modes.
  b. Assesses the stimuli for those behaviors and categorized them as focal, contextual or residual stimuli.
  c. Make statement or nursing diagnosis of the individual's adaptive state.
  d. Set goals to promote adaptation.
  e. Implements interventions aimed at managing the stimuli to promote adaptation of the client.
  f. Evaluates whether the adaptive goals have been met.
- By manipulating the stimuli and not the client the nurse enhance the interaction of the individual with their environment thereby promoting health.
- Senesac (2003) reported that the Roy's adaptation model can be used by individual nurse to understand, plan, and direct nursing practice in the care of individual patients.
- Villarreal (2003) applied the Roy adaptation model in caring of young women who were contemplating smoking cessation.
- Newman (1997) used the Roy adaptation model to caregivers of chronically ill family members.

Nursing Education

- Roy's adaptation model distinguishes nursing science from medical science by having the content of these areas taught in separate courses.
- Roy stresses collaboration with nurse and physician but delineates separate goals for nursing and physicians.
- Roy suggests this model helps to clarify objectives, identifies content and specifies patterns for teaching and learning.
- This model provides nursing educators, a systemic way of teaching students to assess and care for patients within the context of their lives rather than just as victims of illness.
- In the early 1980's the School of Nursing at the University of Ottawa experienced a major curriculum change, i.e. incorporating a nursing model by which to base their new curriculum. They included Roy adaptation model in the first year of the baccalaureate program.

Nursing Research

- Roy adaptation model has been used to guide knowledge development through nursing research.
- Young-McCaughan (2003) by using Roy's adaptation model studied the effect of a structured aerobic exercise tolerance, sleep patterns and quality of life in patients with cancer.

- Bournaki (1997) by using Roy's adaptation model studied pain-related responses to venipuncture in school-age children.
- This model was a useful guide for the design and conduct of studies of functional status.

Limitation

- Theory is very conceptual so it is difficult to understand.
- Four adaptive modes have unclear boundaries.
- Person is good and is to be highest good to be achieved this concept limits its view.

Critique of the Theory

- *Clarity:* Roy's arrangement of concepts is logical, but that the development of definitions is inadequate related to her original format.
- *Simplicity:* This model is complex because has several major concepts and sub concepts, and also has numerous relational statements.
- *Generality:* This theory is generalizable to all settings in nursing practice, but is limited in scope because it primarily addresses the concept of person-environment adaptation and focuses primarily on the client. Information on the nurse is indirect.
- *Empirical precision:* Testable hypothesis
- *Derivable consequences:* It has a clearly defined nursing process and can be useful in clinical practice; and also capable of generating new information through hypothesis testing.

 CLINICAL APPLICATION OF ROY'S ADAPTATION MODEL

Demographic Data of the Client

Name	:	Mr. Kumar
Age	:	58 years
Sex	:	Male
IP number	:	M2863
Education	:	Post graduate
Occupation	:	Bank officer
Marital status	:	Married
Religion	:	Hindu
Informants	:	Client and Wife
Date of admission	:	04/04/2015
Diagnosis	:	Diabetes mellitus

FIRST LEVEL ASSESSMENT

Physiologic-Physical Mode

Oxygenation

- His ventilation and gas exchange is stable.
- Respiratory rate = 20 bpm.
- His chest is in normal shape and chest expansion normal on both sides.
- Air entry equal in bilaterally.
- No abnormal lung sounds like ronchi or crepitus heard.
- S1& S2 sound heard.
- No abnormal heart sounds heard.
- His capillary refill time delayed.
- Apex beat felt and it is normal in rhythm, depth and rate.
- Dorsalis pedis pulsation of affected limp is not palpable.
- His all other pulsations are normal in rate, depth, tension with regular rhythm.
- Blood pressure-110/180 mm Hg.
- Peripheral pulses felt and found normal in rate and rhythm, no clubbing or cyanosis.

Nutrition

- He is on diabetic diet (1500 kcal) since 10 years.
- He is a nonvegetarian.
- His weight reduced recently (12 kg/6 month).
- Digestive process is stable.
- He has complaints of anorexia since last few months.
- He has no abdominal distension, soft on palpation and no tenderness on palpation.
- No visible peristaltic movements.
- Heard bowel sound.
- Dullness over hepatic area on percussion.
- Normal Oral mucosa.
- No difficulty to swallow food

Elimination

- No signs of infections found.
- No pain during micturition or defecation.
- Normal bladder pattern.
- He is using urinal for micturition.
- He complaints of constipation since 3 days.

Activity and Rest

- He is taking adequate rest.
- Due to unfamiliar surroundings sleep pattern disturbed at night.
- He likes to watch movies and interested in reading.
- Not interested in regular pattern of exercise.
- Only he is walking from home to office during morning and evening.
- Activity reduced now due to amputated right leg.
- He is walking with the help of crutches.
- He complaints pain on joints but no swelling and contractures.
- ROM is limited in the right leg due to wound, so he needs assistance for doing his activities.

Protection

- His right lower fore foot is amputated.
- Black discoloration present over the area.
- No redness, discharge or other signs of infection. Temperature: 37 °C
- Wound healing is occurring better now.
- Walking with the use of leg is not possible. So walking with the help of crutches.
- While walking, he complaints of pain on knee and hip joint present.
- Dorsalis pedis pulsation, not present over the right leg. Left leg is normal in length and size.
- Over the foot several papules present.
- All his peripheral pulses are present with normal rate, rhythm and depth over left leg.

Senses

- He has no pain sensation in the wound site.
- Because of neuropathy, he has reduced touch and pain sensation in the lower periphery.
- For reading he is using spectacle.
- Auditory, olfaction, and gustatory senses are normal.

Fluids and Electrolytes

- Drinks approximately 2200 ml of water.
- Stable intake/output ratio.
- Serum electrolyte values are within normal limit.
- No signs of acidosis or alkalosis.
- His blood glucose elevated (FBS: 300 mg/dl).

Neurological Function

- He is conscious and oriented.
- He is very anxious about the disease condition and his future.
- He is showing signs of stress.
- Due to amputation touch and pain sensation decreased in lower extremity.
- His thinking and memory is intact.

Endocrine function

- Due to DM he is on insulin since 9 years.
- Except elevated blood sugar value, no other signs and symptoms of endocrine disorders
- No glands enlarged.

Self-Concept Mode

Physical Self

- He is very anxious about body image changes, but he is accepting treatment and trying to cope with the situation.
- He deprived of sexual activity after amputation of right leg.
- He belongs to a nuclear family (4 members).
- He stays along with wife and two children.
- He is maintaining good relationship with the neighbors and friends.
- He is fairly active in social activities.

Personal Self

- Because of financial burden and hospitalization, self-esteem disturbed.
- He believes in God and worshiping Hindu traditions.

Role Performance Mode

- He was the only earning member in his family. His role shift is not compensated. His son does not have any work. His role clarity is not achieved.

Interdependence Mode

- He is maintaining good relationship with the neighbors, friends, and relatives.
- But he believes, no one is able to help him at this moment.
- He was fairly active in social activities.

Second Level Assessment

Focal Stimulus

- Non-healing wound after amputation of great and second toe of right leg (3 week). A wound first found on the junction between first and second toe 3 month back. The wound was non-healing and gradually increased in size with pus collected over the area.
- He first consulted in a local hospital in his area. From there, they referred to tertiary hospital; where he was admitted for 1 month and 1 week. During hospital stay his right leg's great and second toe amputated. But surgical wound turned to nonhealing with pus and black color. So the surgeon suggested for below knee amputation of right leg. That made them to come to his present hospital. He underwent a plastic surgery 2 week before.

contextual Stimuli

- He is a known case diabetes mellitus for past 12 years.
- He was on oral hypoglycemic agent for initial 3 years.
- But he is switched to insulin and using it for 9 years now.
- He is not wearing foot wear in house and premises.

Residual Stimuli

- He had tuberculosis attack 5 year back, and took complete course of DOT treatment. Previously, he admitted in a hospital for leg pain about 3 year back. Mother had history of PTB. He is a post graduate in economics, so no special knowledge regarding health matters.

CONCLUSION

Mr Kumar was suffering with diabetes mellitus for past 12 years. Right leg diabetic foot ulcer and recent amputation made his life more stressful. Nursing care of this client based on Roy's adaptation model provided had a dramatic change in his condition. His wounds started healing and he planned to discharge on 15th June. He learned how to use crutches and mobilized at least thrice in a day. Client's anxiety reduced to a great extends by proper explanation and reassurance by the care giver (nurse). He gained good knowledge on various aspect of diabetic foot ulcer for the future self-care activities.

Nursing Care Plan

Assessment of behavior	Assessment of stimuli	Nursing diagnosis	Goal	Intervention	Evaluation
Ineffective sense and protection in physical-physiological mode (no pain sensation on the wound site)	Focal stimuli: Non-healing wound after amputation of great and second toe of right leg-3 week	1. Impaired skin integrity related to fragility of the skin secondary to vascular insufficiency	**Long-term objective:** 1. Amputated area will be totally healed by June 2015 2. Skin will remain intact with no ulcerations. **Short-Term Objective:** 1. Size of wound decreases 2. No signs of infection over the wound within 5 days 3. Normal WBC values within 5 days 4. Presence of healthy granular tissues in the wound site within 5 days	• Maintain the wound area clean and dry • Maintain sterile technique while providing cares to the wound to prevent infection • Do wound dressing with betadine solution which promote healing and growth of new tissue. • Check for signs and symptoms of infection or also delay in healing. • Administer the antibiotics prescribed and vitamin C supplementation to enhance the healing process.	**Short-term goal:** MET: • Wound size decreased to less than 1x1 cms. • WBC values became normal gradually **Long-term goal:** Partially Met: • Skin moderately intact with no ulcera tions. • Continue plan re-evaluate goal and interventions • Unmet: Complete healing of amputated area not achieved. Continue plan re-evaluate goal and interventions

Contd...

Contd...

Assessment of behavior	Assessment of stimuli	Nursing diagnosis	Goal	Intervention	Evaluation
Impaired activity in physical-physiological mode	Focal stimuli: During hospital stay great and second toe of right leg amputated. But surgical wound turned is not healed and became pus and black color.	2. Impaired physical mobility related to amputation of the right forefoot and presence of unhealed wound	**Long-term objective:** Patient will attain maximum possible physical mobility within 4 months. **Short-term objective:** 1. Correct use of crutches by June 2015 2. Walking with minimum support by June 2015 3. He will be self-motivated in activities by June 2015	• Assess the level of restriction of his movement • Encourage to do active and passive exercises to all the extremities to improve his muscle tone and strength. • Make the client to do the range of motion exercises to lower extremities which will strengthen his muscle. • Rub the upper and lower extremities which help to improve his circulation. • Provide articles near to the him and encourage to do activities within limits which promote feeling of well being to him. • Provide positive reinforcement for even a small improvement to increasc the frequency of the desired activity. • Pain relief measures should be taken before doing the activities and initiated as pain can hinder with the activity.	**Short-term goal:** Met: He used crutches correctly by June 2015. He is also motivated self in doing minor exercise. Partially Met: he is now walking with minimum support. **Long-term goal:** Unmet: He is not achieved maximum possible physical mobility. Continue plan re-evaluate goal and interventions

Contd...

Contd…

Assessment of behavior	Assessment of stimuli	Nursing diagnosis	Goal	Intervention	Evaluation
Alteration in Physical self in Self-concept mode (He is very nervous about changes in body image) Change in Role performance mode. (He was the only earning member in his family. So his role shift is not compensate)	Contextual stimuli: He is known case diabetes mellitus for past 12 years and on treatment with insulin for 9 years. Residual stimuli: He has no special knowledge in health related matters	3. Anxiety related to hospital admission and unknown outcome of the disease and financial constrains.	**Long-term objective:** The patient will remain free from anxiety. **Short-term objective:** 1. Demonstrating effective coping in the treatment 2. Being able to take rest and sleep 3. Asking less questions	• Allow and encourage him and family to ask questions. • Allow him and his family to verbalize their anxiety. • Provide comfortable and quiet environment for the patient and family	**Short-term goal:** Met: Demonstrated effective coping with treatment. He is able to rest and sleep quietly. **Long-term goal:** Unmet: He is not totally remained free from anxiety due to financial constrains. Continue plan re-evaluate goal and interventions.
	Contextual stimuli: He is a known case diabetes mellitus for past 12 years and on treatment with insulin for 9 years. Residual stimuli: He has no special knowledge in health related matters	4. Deficient knowledge regarding diabetes and its complication the foot care, wound care, diabetic diet, and need of follow up care.	**Long-term objective:** Client will acquire adequate knowledge regarding the diabetes and its complication, foot care, wound care, diabetic diet, and need of follow up care and practice them in their day to day life.	• Explain the treatment measures to the client and their benefits in a understandable language. • Explain about the home care. Include the points like care of foot, wounds, nutrition, activity etc. • Clear the doubts of the client as the client may present with some matters of importance.	**Short-term goal:** Met: demonstration of wound care. Strictly following diabetic diet plan Unmet: Demonstration of foot care. **Long-term goal:** Unmet: He is not completely achieved and practiced

Contd…

Contd…

Assessment of behavior	Assessment of stimuli	Nursing diagnosis	Goal	Intervention	Evaluation
			Short-term objective: 1. Demonstrati-on of foot care effectively. 2. Strictly following diabetic diet plan 3. Also Demonstration of wound care.	• Repeat the information whenever essential to strengthen knowledge.	the necessary knowledge. Continue plan re-evaluate goal and interventions

CONCLUSION

Sister Callista Roy developed the Roy Adaptation Model in Nursing, a theory developed to help nurses in their practice through the understanding of clients as person striving to maintain balance between systems and the outside environment. She says 'My theory will never will be completed, never finished. Knowledge needs to keep developing.'

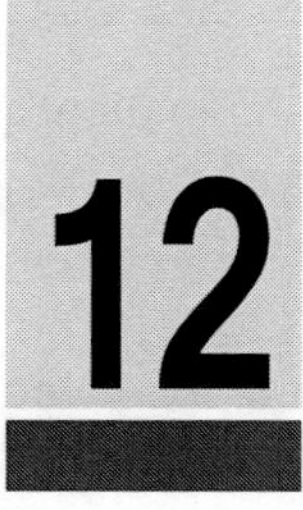

12 Joyce Travelbee: Human to Human Relationship Model

 INTRODUCTION

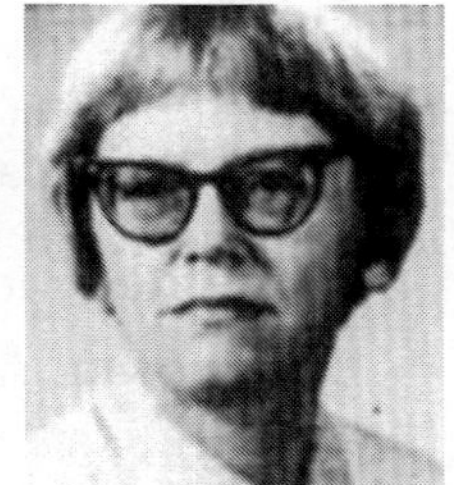
Joyce Travelbee

The theory mainly focuses on the human relationship which is the essence of nursing. The nursing care can be only achieved through maintaining effective therapeutic relationship with patients.

Biography

- She was born in 1926.
- She completed her BSN Degree at Louisiana State University in 1956 and her Master of Science Degree in Nursing at Yale University in 1959.
- Her area of interest and training is Psychiatric Nursing while she was appointed as an instructor at Depaul Hospital Affiliated School, New Orleans.
- She had many research publications and had published a book titled on *Interpersonal Aspects of Nursing* during her service.
- She started a Doctoral program in Florida in 1973. Unfortunately, Travelbee was unable to finish the program due to a brief illness that resulted in her tragic death at the age of 47.

Major Concepts

Suffering, which is 'an experience that varies in intensity, duration and depth...a feeling of unease, ranging from mild, transient mental, physical or mental discomfort to extreme pain....'

Meaning, which is the reason attributed to a person.

Hope, which is a faith that can and will be a change that would bring something better with it. Six important characteristics of hope are: Dependence on other people, future orientation, escape routes, the desire to complete a task or have an experience, confidence that others will be there when needed, and the acknowledgment of fears and moving forward toward its goal.

Communication, which is 'a strict necessity for good nursing care.'

Self-therapy, which is the ability to use one's own personality consciously and in full awareness in an attempt to establish relatedness and to structure nursing interventions. This refers to the nurse's presence physically and psychologically.

Targeted intellectual approach by the nurse toward the patient's situation.

Human-to-Human Relationship Model

According to this model the nurse and the patient undergoes the following series of interactional phases:

- *Original encounter:* The first impression by the nurse of the sick person and *vice-versa.*
- *Emerging identities:* The nurse and patient perceiving each other as unique individuals and the link of relationship begins to form.
- *Empathy:* The ability to share in the person's experience. The result of the emphatic process is the ability to expect the behavior of the individual whom he or she empathized.
- *Sympathy* which happens when the nurse wants to lessen the cause of the patient's suffering.
- *Rapport* is that nursing intervention that lessens the patient's suffering.

Metaparadigm in Nursing

Person: A human being is a unique and irreplaceable individual who is in the continuous process of becoming, evolving and changing.

Health: A person has both subjective and objective health. ' A person's subjective health status is an individually defined state of well-being in accord with self-appraisal of physical-emotional-spiritual status.' Objective health is 'an absence of discernible disease, disability, or defect as measured by physical examination, laboratory tests, assessment by a spiritual director or psychological counselor.'

Environment: Environment was not clearly defined. However, she defined human conditions and life experiences encountered by all men as sufferings, hope, pain, and illness. These conditions are associated to the environment.

Nursing 'an interpersonal process whereby the professional nurse practitioner assists an individual, family or community to prevent or cope with the experience of illness and suffering and, if necessary, to find meaning in these experiences.'

Application of Human-to-Human Relationship Model

Nursing education: This model has been used in different nursing programs and has acted as a guide for nursing students to understand about the health and illness.

Nursing practice: This theory has wide application especially in hospice care where the nurses use to develop rapport and trusting relationship with patient and relatives. According to her it is the onus of a hospice nurse to make understand her patient about the meaning of his death before he begins to accept his death.

Nursing research: Various studies have conducted on the basis of this model and found empirically precise especially in cancer patients.

Critique of the Human-to-Human Relationship Model

Clarity: The concepts are clear, however some of the definitions are repeating.

Simplicity: Simple to understand as it focuses on the patient and nurse interactions.

Generality: Can applicable to only those patients who are in any distress.

Empirical precision: This theory has applied in many researches, though certain concepts are yet to prove as empirically precise.

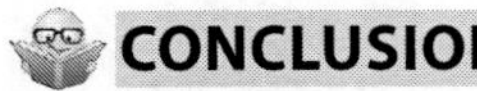

CONCLUSION

Nursing is accomplished through relationships between humans beginning with an original encounter and then progressing through stages of emerging identities, developing feelings of empathy and sympathy.

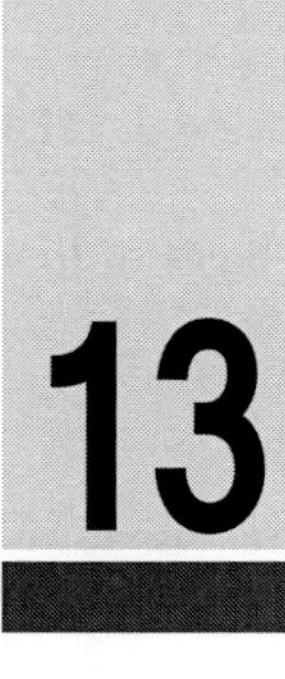

13 Jean Watson: Theory of Caring

'I emphasize that it is possible to read, study, learn about, even teach and research the caring theory; however, to truly 'get it,' one has to personally experience it; thus the model is both an invitation and an opportunity to interact with the ideas, experiment with and grow within the philosophy, and living it out in one's personal/professional life.'

– Jean Watson

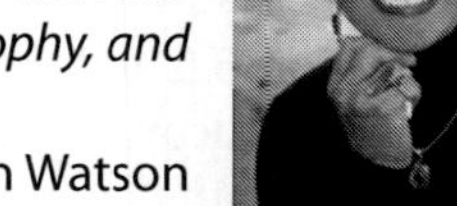

INTRODUCTION

Caring is the integral part of nursing profession. Most of the individuals choose nursing as a profession because of their wish to care for other individuals. In Jean Watson's view, the disease might be cured, but illness would remain because without caring, health is not attained. Several caring theories are developed in nursing, among them, two well known theories were developed in the 1970's, Leininger's Theory of cultural care and Jean Watson's Theory of human caring.

BIOGRAPHY AND ACHIEVEMENTS

- Margaret Jean Harman Watson was born in southern West Virginia and during the 1940s and 1950s in the small town of Welch, Appalachian Mountains of West Virginia.
- She was the youngest of eight children of her parents.
- In 1961 she graduated from the Lewis Gale School of Nursing in Roanoke, Virginia.
- She completed her Bachelor's Degree in nursing in 1964 from University of Colorado at Boulder.
- She received her master of science in nursing in psychiatric and mental health nursing in 1966 from University of Colorado at Boulder.
- She received PhD in educational psychology and counseling in 1973 from University of Colorado at Boulder.
- She lost of her left eye in an accident in 1997 and lost of her husband of 37 years in 1998.
- She is a distinguished Professor of Nursing and holds a Chair in Caring Science at the University of Colorado Health Sciences Center.
- She is a Fellow of the American Academy of Nursing.

- She was a Dean of Nursing at the University Health Sciences Center and President of the National League for Nursing.
- Undergraduate and graduate degrees in nursing and psychiatric-mental health nursing and PhD in educational psychology and counseling.
- She is the founder of the original Center for Human Caring in Colorado and is a Fellow of the American Academy of Nursing.
- In 1988, she published the theory in 'Nursing: Human science and human care'.

Assumptions

- Caring can be successfully demonstrated and practiced only interpersonally.
- Caring consists of carative factors that result in the satisfaction of certain human needs.
- Effective caring promotes health and individual or family growth. Caring can directly contribute to the overall welfare of the individual and his/her family.
- Caring responses accept person not only as he or she is now but as what he or she may become. The potential of an individual is important as the individual in their current state of being.
- A caring environment is one that offers the development of potential while allowing the person to choose the best action for himself or herself at a given point in time. Individual feel more cared for when they are empowered to make their own choices about health care.
- Caring is more 'healthogenic' than is curing. A science of caring is complementary to the science of curing. Caring and curing need to coexist for the people to achieve their maximum health potential.
- The practice of caring is the center of nursing.

METAPARADIGM OF THE THEORY

Dr Watson defines metaparadigm concepts in nursing including person or human being, health, and nursing. They are defined as follows:

- *Human being:* According to Watson, the human being is a valued person, cared for, respected and viewed in a holistic way, as body, mind, and spirit.
- *Health:* Dr Watson believes that there are other factors that are needed to be added in the WHO definition of health. She adds the following three elements:
  - A high level of overall physical, mental and social functioning
  - A general adaptive-maintenance level of daily functioning
  - The absence of illness (or the presence of efforts that leads its absence).
- *Nursing:* She states nursing as a human science of persons and health-illness experience that are mediated by professional, personal, scientific, and ethical care interactions.

- *Environment/Society:* According to Watson 'Caring (and nursing) has existed in every society. Every society has had some people who have cared for others. A caring attitude is not transmitted from generation to generation by genes. It is transmitted by the culture of the profession as a unique way of coping with its environment.'

CONCEPTS OF THE THEORY

The major conceptual elements of the theory are the following:

- *Ten Carative Factors:* Spiritual, emotional, and human care-giving factors that are added to, and meshed with, clinical care factors.
- *A transpersonal caring relationship:* The nurse and client mutually search for meaning and wholeness.
- *Caring moments/caring occasion:* Uninterrupted time spent with a client to make a human-to-human connection.
- **Caring-healing modalities:**

  According to Dr. Watson, the main underpinnings of her theory include carative factors, transpersonal caring relationship and caring occasion/caring moment.

  Other dynamic aspects of the theory that have emerged or are emerging as more explicit components include:
- Expanded views of self and person (transpersonal mind-body-spirit unity of being, embodied spirit).
- Caring-healing consciousness and intentionality to care and promote healing caring consciousness as energy within the human environment field of a caring moment.
- Phenomenal field/unitary consciousness: Unbroken wholeness and connectedness of all.
- Advanced caring-healing modalities/nursing arts as future model for advanced practice of nursing qua nursing (consciously guided by one's nursing ethical-theoretical-philosophical orientation).

Ten Carative Factors

- The original work (Watson, 1979) was based 10 carative factors as a framework for providing a format and focus for nursing phenomena. Although carative factors are still the current terminology for the 'core' of nursing, providing a structure for the initial work. She has extended carative to caritas and caritas processes as consistent with a more fluid and contemporary movement of these ideas and with my expanding directions.
- Caritas comes from the Latin word meaning '*to cherish and appreciate, giving special attention to, or loving.*' It connotes something that is very fine; indeed, it is precious.
- **The 10 carative factors included in the original work are the following**:
  1. Formation of a humanistic-altruistic system of values.

2. Instillation of faith-hope.
3. Cultivation of sensitivity to one's self and to others.
4. Development of a helping-trusting, human caring relationship.
5. Promotion and acceptance of the expression of positive and negative feelings.
6. Systematic use of a creative problem-solving caring process.
7. Promotion of transpersonal teaching-learning.
8. Provision for a supportive, protective, and/ or corrective mental, physical, societal, and spiritual environment.
9. Assistance with gratification of human needs.
10. Allowance for existential-phenomenological-spiritual forces.

- The first three carative factors form the 'philosophical foundation' for the science of caring. The remaining seven carative factors spring from the foundation laid by these first three.
- Some of the basic views of the original carative factors still hold and indeed are used as the basis for some theory-guided practice models and research. She in 2006 as part of her evolution and the evolution of these ideas and the theory itself is to transpose the carative factors into 'clinical caritas processes.'

FROM CARATIVE FACTORS TO CLINICAL CARITAS PROCESSES

Nursing interventions related to human care initially referred to as **carative factors** have now been changed into **clinical caritas processes** (Watson in 2006):

- *The formation of a humanistic-altruistic system of values* becomes: 'practice of loving-kindness and equanimity within context of caring consciousness.'
  - This value system begins to form developmentally at an early age of life and the values shared with the parents.
  - This is can achieve through one's own life experiences, the learning one gains and exposure to the humanities.
  - According to her humanistic values are the basic for caring.
  - Examination of one's own views, beliefs, interaction with various cultures, and personal growth experiences, etc. are help to develop altruistic behavior.
  - These are all perceived as necessary to the nurse's own maturation, which then promotes altruistic behavior toward others.
- *The instillation of faith-hope* becomes: 'Being authentically present, and enabling and sustaining the deep belief system and subjective life world of self and one being cared for.'
  - According to Watson the nurse's role is to promote wellness and positive health through developing effective nurse-patient interrelationships and helping the patient learn how to develop

  health-seeking behaviors. It is necessary for both the carative and the curative processes.
  - The nurse can continue to use faith-hope to provide a sense of well-being through beliefs which are meaningful to the individual, when modern science has nothing further to offer to that client.
- *The cultivation of sensitivity to one's self and to others* becomes: 'Cultivation of one's own spiritual practices and transpersonal self, going beyond ego self.'
  - The nurse and the client achieve self actualization and self acceptance when they recognize the feelings.
  - The nurses realize and accept their own sensitivity and feelings; they become more genuine, authentic and sensitive to others. This help the nurse to explore the need to begin to feel an emotion as it presents itself. It is achieved through development of one's own feeling is needed to interact genuinely and sensitively with others.
  - Strive to become more sensitive, makes the nurse more authentic, which encourages self-growth and self-actualization, in both the nurse and those with whom the nurse interacts.
  - The nurses promote health; when they maintain person to person relationship.
- *The development of a helping-trusting relationship* becomes: 'developing and sustaining a helping-trusting authentic caring relationship.'
  - Strongest tool of the nurse is the mode of communication, which establishes rapport and caring and thereby builds a helping-trust relationship with the client.
  - Characteristics needed to in the helping-trust relationship are: Congruence, Empathy, and warmth
  - Communication includes verbal, nonverbal and listening in a manner which connotes empathetic understanding. For the effective communication , use a moderate speaking volume, open relaxed posture and congruent expression during conversations.
- *The promotion and acceptance of the expression of positive and negative feelings* becomes: 'Being present to, and supportive of the expression of positive and negative feelings as a connection with deeper spirit of self and the one-being-cared-for.'
  - Sharing of feelings is a risky experience for both nurse and client. The nurse must be open and prepared for both positive and negative feelings.
  - 'Feelings alter thoughts and behavior, and they need to be considered and allowed for in a caring relationship.'
  - Awareness of the feelings helps one to understand the behavior it engenders.
- *The systematic use of the scientific problem-solving method for decision making* becomes: 'Creative use of self and all ways of knowing as part of the caring process; to engage in artistry of caring-healing practices.'

   - By using the nursing process; the problem-solving approach dispels the traditional image of the nurse as the doctor's handmaiden.
   - The scientific problem: Solving method is the only method that allows for control and prediction, and that permits self-correction.
- *The promotion of interpersonal teaching-learning* becomes: 'Engaging in genuine teaching-learning experience that attends to unity of being and meaning attempting to stay within other's frame of reference.'
   - The promotion of interpersonal teaching-learning shifts the responsibility of wellness and health to the patient as the nurse facilitates, teaches and enables the patient.
   - The caring nurse must focus on the learning process as much as the teaching process.
   - Understanding the person's perception of the situation help the nurse to prepare a cognitive plan.
- *The provision for a supportive, protective, and (or) corrective mental, physical, socio-cultural, and spiritual environment* becomes: 'creating healing environment at all levels (physical as well as nonphysical), subtle environment of energy and consciousness, whereby wholeness, beauty, comfort, dignity, and peace are potentiated.'
   - Jean Watson divides these into external and internal variables, which the nurse manipulates in order to provide support and protection for the person's mental and physical well-being. The nurse must be aware of the internal and external environment of the client.
   - The external and internal environments are interdependent.
   - Nurse must provide comfort, privacy and safety.
- *Assistance with the gratification of human needs* becomes: assisting with basic needs, with an intentional caring consciousness, administering 'human care essentials,' which potentiate alignment of mind body spirit, wholeness, and unity of being in all aspects of care,' tending to both embodied spirit and evolving spiritual emergence. It is based on a hierarchy of need similar to that of the Maslow's hierarchy of needs.
   - Each need is equally important for quality nursing care and the promotion of optimal health of the client. All the needs of the client deserve to be attended to and valued.
   - The nurse should recognizes the biophysical, psychophysical, psychosocial and intrapersonal needs of self and patient all the while remembering patients must satisfy lower-order needs before attempting to attain higher-order needs.

Watson's (1979) Ordering of Needs:

- *Lower order needs (biophysical needs)-survival needs:*
   - The need for food and fluid
   - The need for elimination
   - The need for ventilation

- *Lower order needs (psychophysical needs)-functional needs:*
  - The need for activity-inactivity
  - The need for sexuality
- *Higher order needs (psychosocial needs)-integrative needs:*
  - The need for achievement
  - The need for affiliation
- *Higher order need (intrapersonal-interpersonal need)-growth-seeking need:*
  - The need for self-actualization.

- *The allowance for existential-phenomenological forces* becomes: 'opening and attending to spiritual-mysterious and existential dimensions of one's own life-death; soul care for self and the one-being-cared-for.'
  - Phenomenology is a way of understanding people from the way things appear to them, from their frame of reference.
  - Existential psychology is the study of human existence using phenomenological analysis.

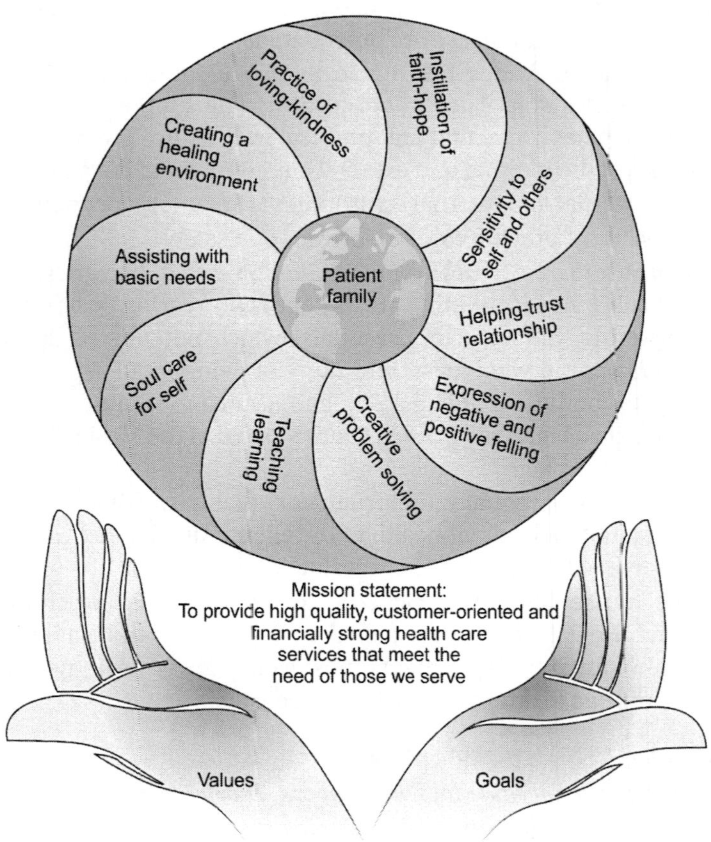

Fig. 13.1: Framework for theory of caring

- This factor helps the nurse to resolve and mediate the incongruity of viewing the person holistically while at the same time attending to the hierarchical ordering of needs.
- Thus the nurse must assist the client to find the strength or courage to meet life or death.
- The nurse has the responsibility to go above and beyond the 10 carative factors and help client to promote their own preventive health actions by teaching patients personal changes to promote health, providing support, teaching problem-solving methods and recognizing coping skills and adaptation to loss.

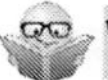 WATSON'S THEORY AND NURSING PROCESS

Watson's nursing process contains the same steps as the scientific research process. These two processes try to solve a problem and provide a framework for decision making.

Assessment

- This phase involves observation, identification and review of the problem; use of applicable knowledge in literature.
- It includes conceptual knowledge for the formulation and conceptualization of framework to assess the problem.
- It also includes the formulation of hypothesis about relationships and defining variables that will be examined in solving the problem.

Plan

- This phase helps to determine how variables would be examined or measured.
- It includes a conceptual approach or design for solving problem and referred as nursing care plan.
- It determines which data should be collected and how on whom.

Intervention

- It is the direct action and implementation of the plan.
- In this phase the collection of the data occurs.

Evaluation

- In this phase analysis of the data as well as the examination of the effects of interventions based on the data occurs.
- It includes the interpretation of the results, the degree to which positive outcome has occurred and whether the result can be generalized.
- It may also generate additional hypothesis or may even lead to the generation of a nursing theory.

LIMITATIONS

- Less important given for biophysical needs of the client.
- The ten carative factors primarily define the psychosocial needs of the person.
- The theory needs further research to apply in practice.
- At moment nurse and client should be present.

APPLICATIONS

Nursing Practice

- Watson's theory has been used in various aspects clinical setting.
- The major concepts of this theory enhance the nurse-patient interaction and improve practice for patients.
- Watson's theory can apply in mental health settings and areas where biophysiological methods of care are no longer as effective, such as in oncology and critical care environments.
- Watson's theory will remain a key factor for all nurses to study and apply as they provide care for their patients, as the population ages and the health care system is more taxed.
- Watson's theory was selected for use in a Hospital called Saint Joseph, in Orange, California state. It is the framework basis of nursing practice in that hospital.
- The theory of Watson is also the recommended because it acts as a guide in patient care for hypertensive clients. This was after a study of the theory relation with quality of the life it contributes to hypertensive clients (Timber, 2009).
- ANNA has approved the theory as it can be used to no more about the dimension of polycystic kidney disease in adults by Martin, LS (1991).

Nursing Education

- Students can use this theory of framework to provide comprehensive care to the clients.
- In USA and other parts of world use Watson's theory based activities as guide to practice.
- By utilizing this theory, nurse educators can help empower nursing students and promote their psychosocial wellness.

Nursing Research

- Still research works are going on based this theory.
- Mullaney, JAB (2000). The lived experience of using Watson's actual caring occasions to treat depressed women.
- Wafika A, Suliman , Elizabeth Welmann, Tagwa Omer, and Laisamma Thomas (2009) were used Watson theory to assess patient perceptions of being cared for in a multicultural environment

 CRITIQUE OF THE THEORY

- *Clarity:* Use of complicated language and lengthy phrases often require multiple readings to gain meaning of the concepts.
- *Simplicity:* Difficult to understand and draws on many disciplines, requiring readers to be familiar with broad subject matter.
- *Generality:* Provides a moral and philosophical basis for all specialties of nursing and this theory focuses more on psychosocial aspects of nursing than on physiological aspects.
- *Empirical precision:* Strengthened by using accepted work from other disciplines, research works are going on.

PRACTICAL APPLICATION OF WATSON'S THEORY OF CARING

Mrs Seema, 60 years old who is admitted to the cardiac department with diagnosis of myocardial infarction. The nurse is familiar with her because she was taking care of Mrs Seema when she previously admitted with the same diagnosis *(caritas processes 4).* The nurse has always liked and appreciated this patient *(caritas processes 1).* The nurse received the patient on the day she is admitted. She gives faint smile to the nurse. The nurse inquire about how she is fairing on and remembered her about her previous creative means that would help her to comply with her prescription *(caritas processes 6 and 7).* As the nurse was previously take care of Mrs. Seema, she is aware of nurse commitment to taking good care her through her suffering *(caritas processes 4).* From her faint smile the nurse come to know about her depression that she is again admitted with the same disease. The nurse begins to talk to her and understand about her perceptions and her lived experiences *(caritas processes 3, 5 and 10).*The nurse helped her to settle in her room and make up surroundings for her to relax *(caritas processes 8).* By the time the nurse inquire more on how she feels now, about her priorities of care and also generally about her *(caritas processes 5 and 10).* The nurse assisted her to go to the toilet *(caritas processes 9)*. She tells to the nurse that she won't et social importance and recognition she used to have before. (It is important to see beyond the physical body of somebody and to focus on the soul and mind).

The nurse told her that she will visit her later as she sensed that the patient like to be alone for some time. The nurse closed the door to ensure her privacy and comfort *(caritas processes 8)*. To promote hope in Mrs. Seema especially when their state is sad can be overwhelming *(caritas processes 2)*. However, because nurse believe that inspiring hope is very important in restoring harmony in her, she has to be creative enough *(caritas processes 6)*. To care for her is very important to nurse as through it she can achieve her motivation, which improves the way she conceptualize herself in her profession.

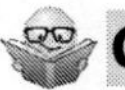

CONCLUSION

This is a theory which given more importance to the caring. Dr. Watson provides many concepts which can be used in many practices. Watson's theory of Human Caring, and the ten Caritas Processes, is one of the prominent theories used in many of the magnet systems. This theory incorporates a holistic approach to patient care and focuses on the relationship between the patient and nurse.

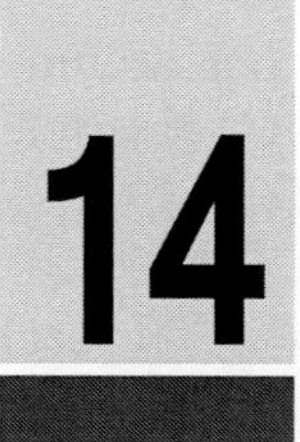

14 Ernestine Wiedenbach: Prescriptive Theory— A Situation Producing Theory

INTRODUCTION

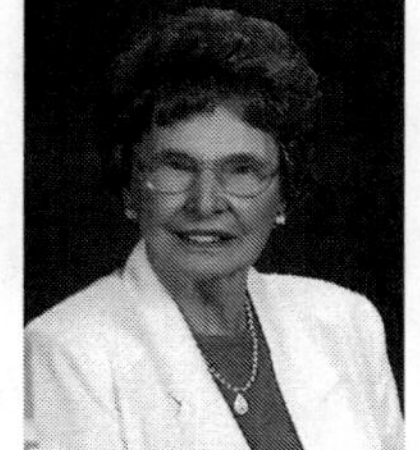

Ernestine Wiedenbach

According to this theory all the nursing actions must be toward an achievement of a goal which consists of these elements; central purpose, prescriptions, and realities.

Biography

- Born in 1900 in Hamburg, Germany.
- In 1925 she received registered nurse diploma from Johns Hopkins Hospital School of Nursing.
- In 1934, received a master's degree and a Certificate in Public Health Nursing from Teachers College, Columbia University.
- Graduated with a certificate in nurse-midwifery from the Maternity Center Association School for Nurse-Midwives in New York History in 1946.
- She started to work as an instructor in maternity Nursing at Yale University in 1952, eventually to an Assistant and Associate professor I Obstetric Nursing in 1954 and 1956 respectively.
- Published her book titled '*Family-Centered Maternity Nursing*' in 1958.
- She left this world on March 8, 1988.

Major concepts: Her theory is mainly influenced by three factors central purpose, prescriptions and realities.

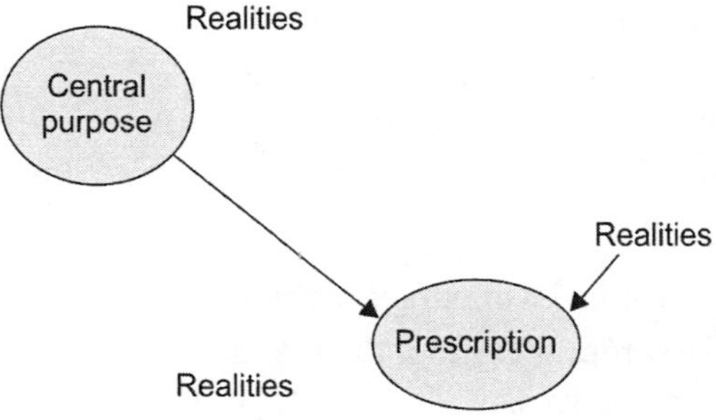

Fig. 14.1: Factors influencing nursing action

The central purpose or philosophy: The nurses' philosophy is their attitude and belief about life and how that affected reality for them. There essential components associated with a nursing philosophy are:

- Reverence for life
- Respect for the dignity, worth, autonomy and individuality of each human being and
- Resolution to act on personally and professionally held beliefs.

Prescription: are the nursing actions which are based on the purpose. These actions can be voluntary and involuntary and categorized in to three:

- *Mutually understood and agreed upon action:* The recipient understands the implication of the action and is receptive to it.
- *Recipient-directed action:* Recipient directs the way the action is carried out.
- *Practitioner-directed action:* Practitioner carries out the action.

Reality: Immediate situation that influence the fulfillment of the central purpose. The realities are considered after being the central purpose and prescriptions are considered. The main five realities are agent or nurse, patient, goal, activities, and the framework.

Metaparadigm in Nursing

Person: Each person is endowed with a unique potential to develop self-sustaining resources. People generally tend toward independence and fulfillment of responsibilities. Self-awareness and self-acceptance are essential to personal integrity and self-worth.

Health: Not defined clearly by the Ernestine Wiedenbach, however definitions of nursing, patient, and need-for-help, and the relationships among these concepts imply health-related concerns in the nurse-patient situation.

Environment: It is inferred that the environment may produce obstacles resulting in a need-for-help experienced by the person. Wiedenbach does not specifically address the concept of environment.

Nursing: Nursing primarily consists of identifying a patient's need for help. The Art of nursing includes:

- Understanding patients needs and concerns.
- Developing goals and actions intended to enhance patients ability.
- Directing the activities related to the medical plan to improve the patient's condition.

The primary responsibilities of nurses include:

1. To reconcile assumptions about the realities.
2. To specify the objectives.
3. To practice nursing according to the objectives.
4. To engage in related activities that contributes to self-realization and the improvement of nursing.

Steps Involved in Direct Patient Care

Identification: Individualization of patient, his experiences, recognition of perception of his condition.

Ministration: Providing the needed help; requires identification of need-for-help, selection of helping measure appropriate to that need, and acceptability.

Validation: Evidence that the patient's functional ability was restored as a result of the help given.

Application of Prescriptive Theory: A Situation Producing Theory

Nursing education: She proposed the nursing education prepares nursing students to practice their profession. This theory has been the foundation for many nursing programs.

Nursing practice: It is widely applicable in nursing practice today. According to Wiedenbach, the practice of clinical nursing is an 'Overt action, directed by disciplined thoughts and feelings toward meeting the patient's need-for-help.'

Nursing research: There as a shift from focus of nursing research from medical illness to patient's responses to health care experiences. This theory support research designed to promote family relationships, to control factors responsible for disabling conditions, and to foster sound health practices.

Critique of the Prescriptive Theory: A Situation Producing Theory

Clarity: All the concepts in this theory is clear and able to understand.

Simplicity: Though the main idea is concerned about the nursing actions is simple, various concepts are interrelated which has the same meaning.

Generality: The scope of the concepts of patient, nursing, and need-for help are very broad and thus possesses generality. However, i.e. not applicable to the infant, comatose patient or many physiologically or psychologically incompetent persons.

Empirical precision: The concepts in this theory can be operationally defined and measurable.

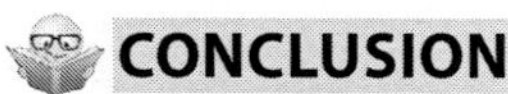

CONCLUSION

The primary focus of nursing is to identification of the patients need and prescriptions of nursing actions on the basis of identified need.

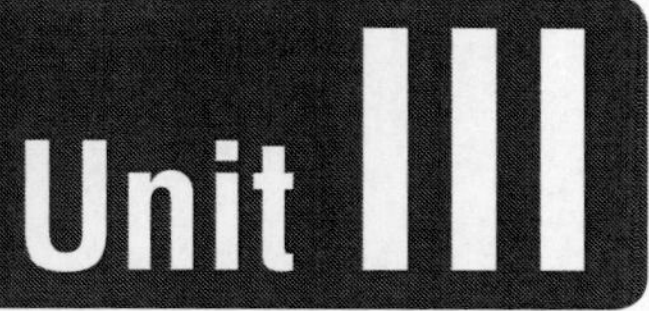

MIDDLE-RANGE NURSING THEORIES

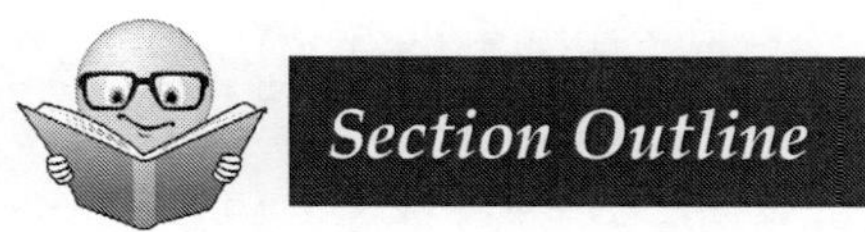

Adam Evelyn: Conceptual Model for Nursing

 INTRODUCTION

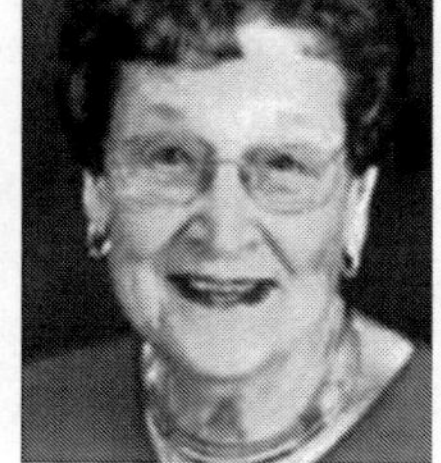
Adam Evelyn

Adam Evelyn a Canadian nurse whose work is primarily focuses on making the concepts and framework for the nursing. This theory differentiates between the conceptual framework and theory.

Biography

- Born in 1929, Ontario Canada.
- In 1950 she received diploma in nursing from hotel Dieu Hospital in Kingston Ontario.
- She graduated from university of Montreal in 1966 and received masters degree in Nursing from University of California in 1971.
- Her first book published in 1971 and later she reprinted its English version in 1991 titled *To Be A Nurse.*
- She published many papers on Conceptual models and theory during her tenure in University of Montreal as teaching faculty.
- She received doctorate in nursing from Laval University, Quebec City in 1992.

Assumptions

- The nurse has a unique function, although she shares certain functions with other professionals.
- When a nurse takes over the physician's role, she delegates her primary function to inadequately prepared personnel.
- Society wants and expects nursing service from the nurse and no other worker is as able or willing to give it.

Major Concepts

Concept is an idea, mental image or can be a generalization formed and developed in the mind. Conceptualization of a reality is known as **conception.**

Conceptual model which is usually based on or derives from a theory and it is not the reality; it is just a mental image of reality or the way of conceptualizing reality. Hence, a conceptual model in nursing is the conception of nursing.

Theory is a system of interrelated prepositions used to describe, predict, explain, understand and control a part of the empirical world.

Needs are the requirement of a human being to maintain health.

Problems are the difficulty or the hurdles arise in the progress toward the health or during the maintenance of health. A *nursing problem* is those problems which require nursing assistance.

Nursing diagnosis is a particular requirements of the patients which cannot be met because insufficient strength and knowledge.

Problem solving methods: The scientific approach which is being used by a professional nurse to solve any problems faced by the clients in a systemic manner.

Helping relationship: The interactions between the patient and nurse to maintain the integrity of the patient. The nurse must have certain qualities, such as empathy, respect; genuine is indispensible to maintain this relationship.

Intervention: The actions which is done by a professionally trained nurse to restore the clients' independence. Each need has biological, physiological, and psychosocial aspects. The nurse complements and supplements the client's strength, knowledge, and will.

Metaparadigm in Nursing

Person: An individual, family or group who possess a particular need on biological, physiological and psychosociocultural dimensions.

Health: Health is not precisely defined by Adam, however she mentioned nursing is primarily focusing to restore the clients' independence.

Environment: Only of the principles which focuses on the environment, but sociocultural dimensions of all the others needs show the environment is an integral part in deciding the client health status.

Nursing: Nurses' role is to make the client independence in the satisfaction of his needs. This can be done by identification of needs, determination of the available resources, planning and interventions of nursing actions, evaluation of effectiveness of nursing interventions with reference to goals.

Application of Adam Evelyn's Conceptual Model for Nursing

Nursing education: On her book she mentioned the objectives, goals and contents of nursing courses. The course content can be official and unofficial. The official content is formally recognized and actually taught, whereas the unofficial contents are not formally taught which is being learned without supervision.

Nursing practice: Nurses help the patient to independence in the satisfaction of his needs by the following steps identification of needs, determination of the available resources, planning and interventions of nursing actions, and evaluation.

Nursing research: This model has been the framework for various nursing researches across the globe.

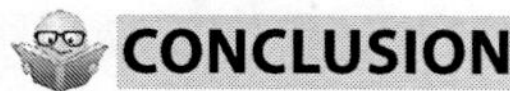

CONCLUSION

Every nurse has to use a conceptual model while rendering nursing care to their patients. This model makes nurses to understand how to use this model through identification of needs, determination of the available resources, planning and interventions of nursing actions, and evaluation.

16 Bennett Mary: PNI Nursing Theory

INTRODUCTION

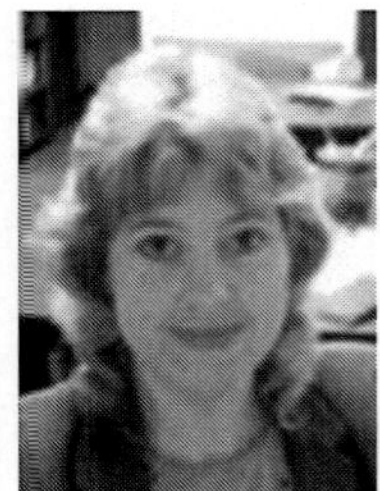

Bennett Mary

The Psychoneuroimmunology Theory Information (PNI) describes the various levels of nursing practice, gives some examples for model implementation at the advanced practice level, and proposes some outcome objectives for model evaluation.

Biography

Assumptions

- There are multidimensional factors which affect well-being, and not all of these factors are physical or genetic.
- Psychosocial factors such as stressful life events, personality traits, and behavioral or lifestyle factors all have an effect upon the person's well-being.
- Socio-environmental factors, such as income, occupation, religion, common social culture, and family all influence a person's health related options and choices that they make.
- Many of these multidimensional factors are capable of being modified by a variety of Therapeutic Nursing Interventions (TNI). (Fig 16.1)

Major Concepts

Psychoneuroimmunology is the basic phenomena of this theory which means interactions between the nervous system and the immune system and the subsequent effects upon disease development and progression.

The model assert that there are many factors which affect well-being, and the effects of many of these factors on wellbeing can be modified by the appropriate use of TNI. These nursing interventions can be holistic, environmental, and traditional.

Holistic interventions: These interventions act to modify the effect of negative stressful life events, psychosocial factors, and behavioral factors upon the PNI network, and thus upon well-being.

Environmental interventions: These endeavors, such as professional activism for quality of care and safe staffing levels, or political activism to improve access to health care, are aimed at improving the health care environment.

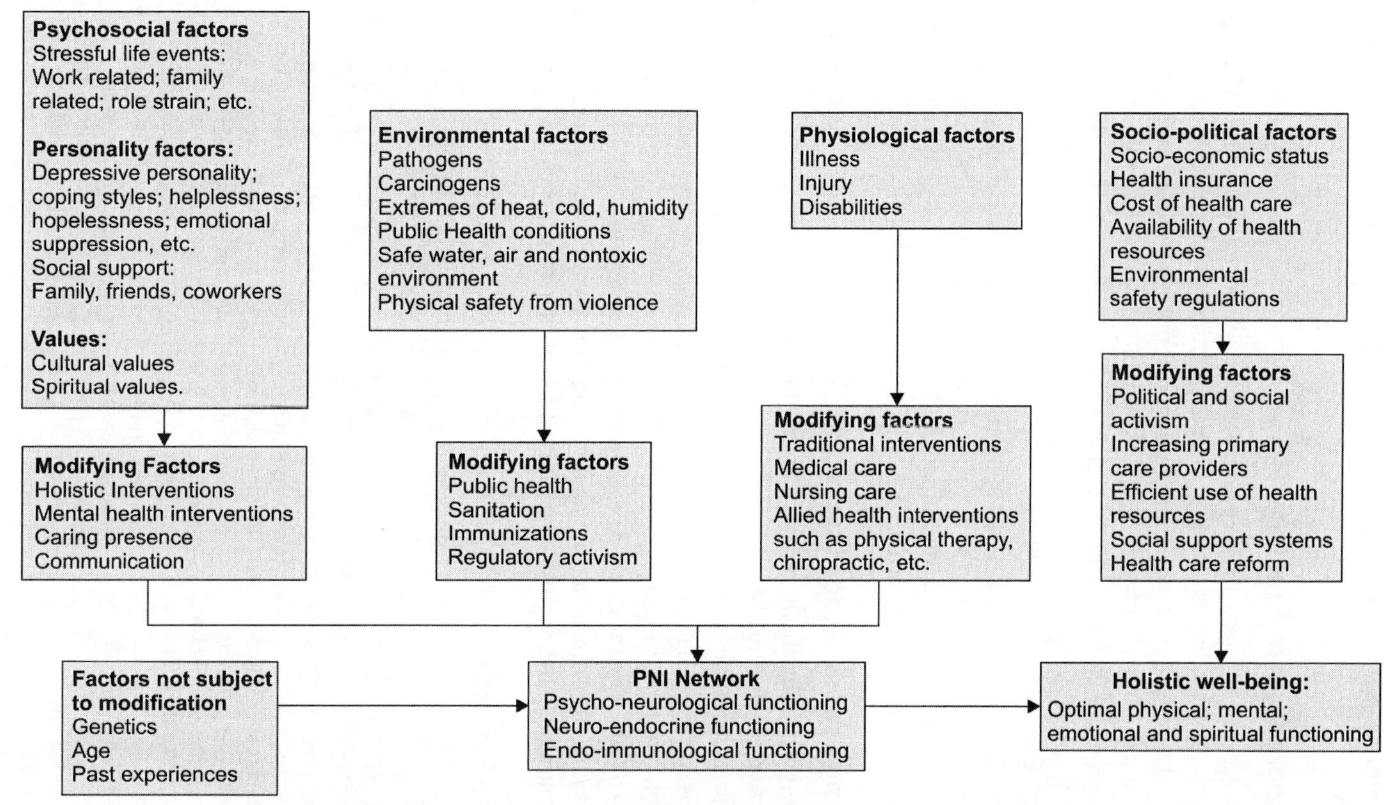

Fig. 16.1: Multidimensional factors affecting well-being: A PNI based model for therapeutic nursing intervention

Traditional interventions: These are aimed at directly improving a client's physical functioning. This may be because most traditional health interventions have been aimed at modifying these physiological factors directly.

Metaparadigm in Nursing

Person: A person or persons with whom the nurse interacts with, and develops TNI for, in order to improve that person(s) health or health environment.

Health: It is the optimal level of physical, mental, emotional and spiritual well-being that the client(s) is capable of at this point in his/her life.

Environment: It is the 'world' in which a client(s) lives, as they themselves view it. A health environment is affected by multi-dimensional factors, many of which can be modified by TNI.

Nursing: The art of using TNI to improve well-being in persons, families and communities. Holistic well-being is achieved by working with clients to devise appropriate and individualized therapeutic nursing interventions, and by helping clients evaluate their own progress towards their goals.

Nursing Process according to PNI

Assessment: Assessment must be focus on the following areas personal, family and environmental.

Diagnosis: Formulation of specific problems based on the assessment.

Therapeutic nursing interventions (TNI): Holistic, environmental, and traditional nursing interventions to achieve the well-being of the client.

Expected outcome: The desired results of nursing interventions.

Evaluation: The outcomes measured include a variety of factors which demonstrate client progress towards optimal well-being.

A Case Scenario

Assessment	Diagnosis	Therapeutic Nursing Interventions (TNI)	Expected Outcomes	Evaluation
27 year woman experiencing unusual thirst, dizziness, blurred vision, and an awkward feeling of numbness in her right foot. Is not taking any medications at this time.	Foot ulcer secondary to diabetes and footwear choices.	Clean foot ulcer and treat with antibiotic ointment. Teach diabetic foot care. Explain the need for good shoes and socks at all times.	No signs and symptoms of infection. Wound healing overtime. Better choices of footwear. Good diabetic foot care.	Wound has healed by second visit one month later. Client wearing walking shoes with cotton socks.

Contd...

Contd...

Assessment	Diagnosis	Therapeutic Nursing Interventions (TNI)	Expected Outcomes	Evaluation
Was wearing sandals without socks at time of assessment. Physical Assessment: Height-5.3. Weight-98 kg Blood pressure-150/96.		Explore client resources and if inadequate, refer to community resources for shoes and socks.		
Family/Cultural Assessment: Lives on the reservation with her parents, her sister, brother and grandfather. Grandfather is in good health, walks frequently and eats a traditional tribal diet, avoiding 'civilized junk food'. Family history of type 2 diabetes. Peer eating customs tend towards high sugar, fat and calorie foods. Sedentary lifestyle, similar to that of other members of her peer group. Not employed.	Obesity related to combined genetics cultural, environ-ment and lifestyle factors.	Explain the relationship between obesity, diabetes and high blood pressure. Work with client to discover better choices in food and exercise that are available to her. Encourage client to work with her family on helping her change to a more traditional tribal diet, high in fiber and low in fat and sugar. Encourage realistic weight loss goals, no more than 1–2 pounds a week, etc.	Decreasing weight over time. Change in exercise levels with increasing aerobic activity overtime. Change in eating habits.	Making good progress towards goals.

CONCLUSION

People make the choices they do because of a variety of factors, such as family values, personal resources and their own environmental situation. All of these factors need to be taken into account when working with the client to develop appropriate TNI to meet their specific needs.

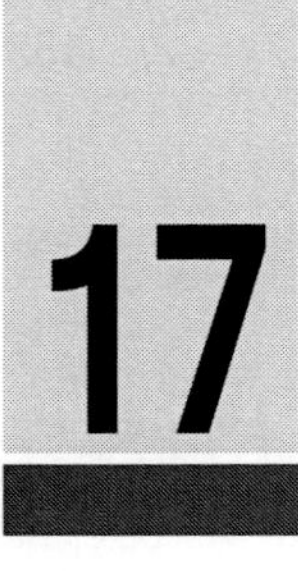

Merle Mishel: Uncertainty in Illness Theory

 INTRODUCTION

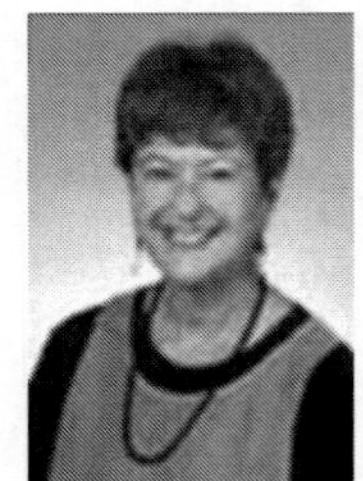
Merle Mishel

This theory explains how uncertainty develops in patients with an acute illness and how patients are proposed to deal with uncertainty.

Biography

- She was born in 1939 in Boston Massachusetts.
- She graduated in 1961 with a Bachelors of Arts from Boston University.
- Master of Science in Psychiatric Nursing from University of California in 1966.
- Received PhD in social psychology from Claremont Graduate school, Claremont California.
- Her areas of research interest are the uncertainty and its management of patient with chronic illness.

Assumptions

- Uncertainty is a cognitive state, representing the inadequacy of an existing cognitive schema to support the interpretation of illness-related events.
- Uncertainty is an inherently neutral experience, neither desirable nor aversive until it is appraised as such.
- Adaptation represents the continuity of an individual's usual biopsychosocial behavior and is the desired outcome of coping efforts to either reduce uncertainty appraised as danger or maintain uncertainty appraised as opportunity.
- Drawing on tenets of chaos theory of people typically function in far-from-equilibrium states.
- A person needs time to focus on self, and if this time is not available, the process of integrating the uncertainty into one's view of life will not occur.

Major Concepts

Stimuli frame: These are the perceived stimuli that are registered into the patient schema. This can be symptom patter, event familiarity and event congruency.

Cognitive capacity: It is the person ability to understand and register information which can be altered with illness.

Structure providers: These are the resources available such as doctors, nurses and other health care professionals to help the patients.

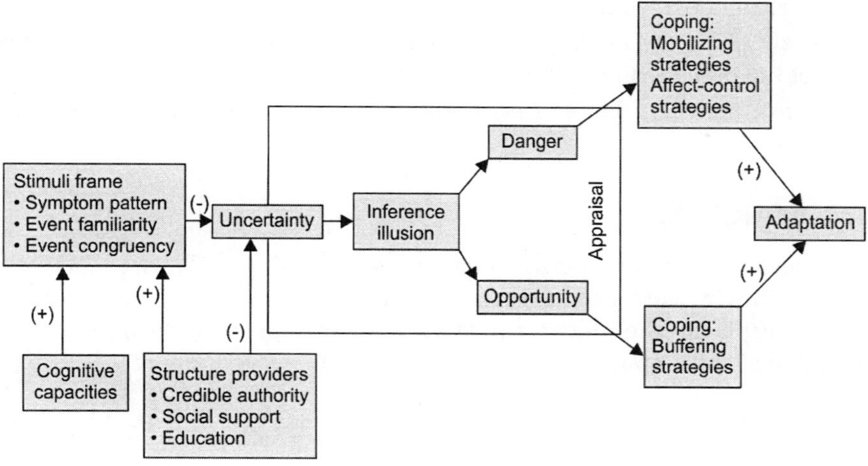

Fig. 17.1: Model of perceived uncertainty in illness

Uncertainty: A situation in which an individual unable to understand the meaning and outcome of the illness associated events.

Cognitive schema: It is an individual perception about the illness, treatment and hospitalization.

Inference: It is the evaluation of situation by patient which can be based on patient experience and knowledge.

Illusion: It is the beliefs which are developed in the patient about uncertainty.

Danger: A situation in which patient experience higher level of uncertainty and poor coping strategies.

Opportunity: The way of living with the uncertainty.

Adaptation: It is the way in which the person is coping with the uncertainty.

Metaparadigm in Nursing

Person: The one who experiences uncertainty gradually, beginning as the illness insidiously invades life.

Health: When an individual build coping styles are moving towards health.

Environment: Illness affects many aspects of the life and importance of influence of environment is yet to be researched.

Nursing: Nurses can assist the patient by constructing a personal scenario for the illness which includes why or how the illness began, how it will progress, and how the patient can recover.

Critique of Uncertainty in Illness Theory

Clarity: Though uncertainty in illness in an abstract concept, this model has presented each concept very clearly.

Simplicity: All the definitions and concepts are very simple, though the complete model is complex.

Generality: This can be used in all areas of nursing practice not only by the nurses but other health care professionals also.

Empirical precision: Limited instruments are available to measure way of copings.

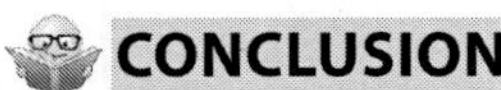

CONCLUSION

The theory explains how persons construct the meaning for illness events with uncertainty indicating the absence of meaning. A model of the uncertainty theory displaying the concepts and their relationships forms the basis for the theoretical and empirical material.

18 Kolcaba K: The Comfort Theory

'I believe the opposite of comfort is suffering.'

–Katharine Koleba

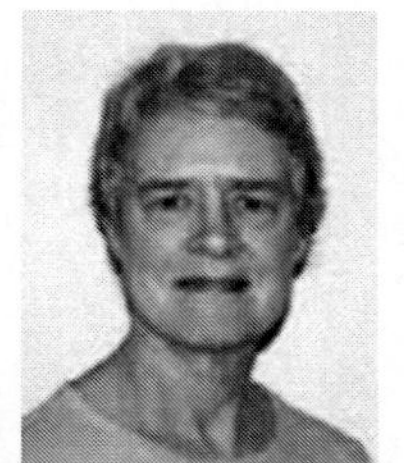

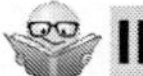 INTRODUCTION

The term comfort is a holistic and complex word. Dr Katharine Kolcaba has been continually advancing and sharing her theory across the spectrum of health care disciplines. With the help of Kolcaba and other health scientists, comfort is re-emerging as a value-added outcome for evidence-based practice. The theory of comfort which is developed in 1990s by Katharine Kolcaba is one of the many middle-range nursing theory because it is focused on a limited dimension of the reality of nursing. It is formulated to provide guidance for nurses in everyday practice and scholarly research rooted in the discipline of nursing.

Biography and Achievements

- She was born on December 8th, 1944 as Katharine Arnold (Kolcaba) in Cleveland, Ohio.
- She received her diploma in nursing in 1965 from St Luke's Hospital School of Nursing.
- In 1987, she completed her graduation from the Frances Payne Bolton School of Nursing, Case Western Reserve University.
- In 1997, she graduated with PhD in Nursing and received certificate of authority clinical nursing specialist.
- In 1997, she developed website called The Comfort Line, http://www.thecomfortline.com
- She is specialized in Gerontology, End of Life and Long Term Care Interventions, Comfort Studies, Instrument Development, Nursing Theory, and Nursing Research.
- She currently working as an associate professor of nursing at Emeritus Status College of Nursing, University of Akron.
- She published Comfort Theory and Practice: A Vision for Holistic Health Care and Research in 2003.

 METAPARADIGM OF KOLCABA'S THEORY

The concepts of metaparadigm as defined by Katharine Kolcaba as follows:

Nursing

- Nursing is considered as the process of assessing comfort needs of the patients, families or communities, and developing and implementing proper nursing interventions, and following nursing interventions patient comfort is evaluated.
- Intentional assessment of comfort needs the design of comfort measures to address those needs. The reassessment of comfort levels after implementation of comfort measures.
- Assessment may be either objective, such as in the observation of wound healing, or subjective, such as by asking the patient that he is comfortable.

Health

- Health is considered to be optimal functioning of the patient, group, family or community facilitated by enhanced comfort.

Person/Patient

- Patients can be considered as individuals, families, institutions, or communities in need of health care including primary, tertiary, or preventive care.

Environment

- Any aspect of the patient, family, or community surroundings that affect comfort and can be manipulated by a nurse(s), or loved one(s) to enhance comfort.

ASSUMPTIONS

According to Kolcaba, the following are the assumptions:
- Individuals have holistic responses to complex stimuli.
- Comfort is a desirable holistic outcome that is germane for the discipline of nursing.
- Individuals strive to meet, or to have met, their basic comfort needs; it is an active endeavor.
- When comfort needs are met, patients are strengthened.
- Institutional integrity has a normative and descriptive component that is based on a patient-oriented value system.

CONCEPTS OF COMFORT THEORY

- Kolcaba first began 'theorizing about the outcome of comfort' while working on a dementia unit as a head nurse and pursuing her Masters of science in Nursing at Case Western Reserve University.

- According to Kolcaba, comfort is the product of holistic nursing art.
- Kolcaba (1994, 2001, 2003) has defined comfort as 'the immediate state of being strengthened through having the human needs for *relief, ease, and transcendence* addressed in four contexts of experience (*physical, psychospiritual, sociocultural, and environmental*)'.
- Kolcaba derived her ideas regarding types of comfort in the concept analysis of three early nursing theorists namely Ida Jean Orlando, Virginia Henderson and Josephine Paterson and Loretta Zderad. These ideas are: *relief*—was derived from the work of Orlando who said that nurses relieved the needs expressed by their patients; *ease*—from the work of Henderson wherein she described the 14 basic functions of human beings to be maintained during care, and *transcendence*—from the work of Paterson and Zderad who proposed that patients rise above their difficulties with the help of nurses.
- **Taxonomic structure of comfort:**
  - According to Kolcaba, types of comfort are:
    - *Relief:* The patient experiences comfort in the sense of relief, if specific comfort needs of a patient are met. For example, a patient who receives antiemetic medication in vomiting feels relief as comfort.
    - *Ease:* Ease addresses comfort in a state of calm and contentment. For example, the patient's anxieties are calmed.
    - *Transcendence:* The state of comfort in which one rises above one's challenges i.e. problems or pain. For example, the patient feels confident about ambulation although he knows it will increase pain.
  - Also Kolcaba describes four contexts in which patient comfort can occur. They are:
    - *Physical:* Kolcaba considered the physical context of comfort as any comfort that pertaining to bodily sensations. For example, positioning, returning to bed when requested and better seating arrangements.
    - *Psychospiritual:* The psychospiritual context of comfort is pertaining to internal awareness of self, including esteem, concept, identity, sexuality, meaning in one's life, and one's relationship to a higher order or being. For example, feeling of satisfaction and fulfillment of ego integrity boosts self-esteem.
    - *Environmental:* Kolcaba described the environmental context of comfort pertaining to external surroundings of the patient, conditions, and influences. For example, a comfortable, safe, and healthy environment promotes an atmosphere of comfort to the patient.
    - *Sociocultural:* The sociocultural context of comfort is defined as pertaining to interpersonal, family, and societal relationships. For

example, culturally sensitive attitudes of nurses towards different cultures and social groups conveys a comforting behavior.

	Relief	Ease	Transcedence
Physical			
Psychospritual			
Environmental			
Sociocultural			

THEORETICAL MODEL

Major concepts and definitions used in conceptual framework are the following:

- *Health care needs:* are those recognized by the patient/family in a particular practice setting or situation.
- *Comforting interventions* are nursing interventions that are considered to address specific comfort needs of recipients. This includes physiological, social, financial, psychological, spiritual, environmental, and physical interventions.
  - Comfort interventions have three categories:
    - *Standard comfort:* Interventions to maintain homeostasis and control pain (e.g. vital signs, lab results, patient assessment, medications and treatment).
    - *Coaching:* To relieve anxiety, provide reassurance and information, instill hope, listen, and help plan for recovery (e.g. emotional support, reassurance, education, listening).
    - *Comfort food for the soul:* Those extra nice things that nurses do to make children/families feel cared for and strengthened, such as massage or guided imagery (e.g. therapeutic touch, music therapy, spending time, personal connections).
- *Intervening variables* Are those factors that are not likely to change and over which providers have little control such as prognosis, financial situation, extent of social support, age, attitude, emotional state, past experience, etc.
- *Enhanced comfort:* According to comfort theory, enhanced comfort is an immediate desirable outcome of nursing care. When comfort interventions are delivered consistently overtime, they are correlated with

a trend toward increased comfort levels overtime, with desired health seeking behaviors (HSBs), and with improved institutional outcomes.

- *Health seeking behavior* (HSBs): The concept of HSBs was first introduced by Schlotfeldt (1975). The relationships between comfort and health seeking behaviors are entailed in the second part of Kolcaba's comfort theory HSBs can be internal behavior, external behavior, or a peaceful death.
  - **Internal behavior:** Healing, immune function, number of T cells, etc.
  - **External behavior:** Health related activities, functional outcomes.
  - **Peaceful death.**
- *Institutional Integrity* (InI): It is defined by Kolcaba (2007) as the values, financial stability, and wholeness of health care organizations at local, regional, state, and national levels. In addition to hospital systems, the definition of 'institutions' includes public health agencies, medicare and medicaid programs, home care agencies, nursing home consortiums, etc. Examples of variables related to this expanded definition of InI include patient satisfaction, cost savings, improved access, decreased morbidity rates, decreased hospitalizations and readmissions, improved health-related outcomes, efficiency of services and billing, and positive cost-benefit ratios. Relationships between comfort, HSBs, and InI constitute the third part of the theory.
  - **Best policies:** They are protocols and procedures developed by an institution for overall use after collecting evidence.

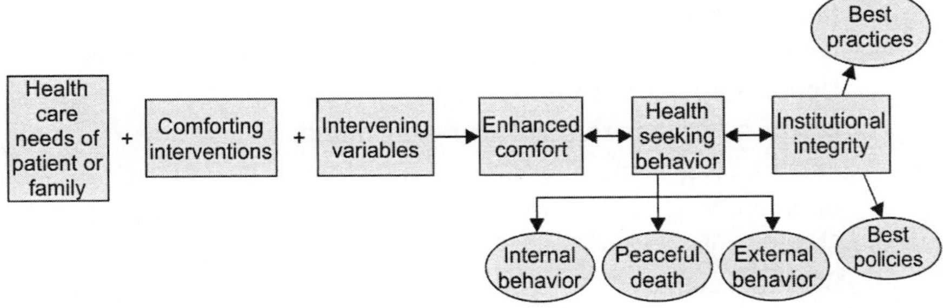

Fig. 18.1: Conceptual framework for comfort theory

Best practices: They are those protocols and procedures developed by an institution for specific patient/family applications (or types of patients) after collecting evidence.

PROPOSITIONS IN KOLCABA'S THEORY OF COMFORT

- Nurses identify the client's comfort needs that have not been met by existing support systems.
- Nurses plan interventions to achieve those needs.
- The intervening variables are taken into account in planning the interventions and mutually agreeing upon reasonable immediate (enhanced comfort) and/or subsequent HSBS outcomes.

- If enhanced comfort is achieved, patients are strengthened to engage in health seeking behaviors or a peaceful death.
- When patients engage in health seeking behaviors more fully, institutions do better and institutions with higher 'integrity' facilitate higher engagement in HSBs.

ENHANCING THE COMFORT OF NURSES

- According to comfort theory, when the comfort of the nurse is enhanced, nurses are more satisfied, more committed to the institution, and also able to work more effectively.
- These better outcomes result in improved patient care and increase institutional strength.
- *Physical comfort:*
  - Safe and clean environment with noise controlled
  - Rest between duty with good tea or coffee
  - Shift duty with adequate leave and off
  - Continuity of patient care
  - Adequate staff
  - Adequate resources and control over them
  - Good wages, benefits and retirement
  - Enough space to work
- *Psychospiritual comfort:*
  - Managerial support
  - Decrease non-nursing work by recruitment of class IV workers
  - Opportunities for advancement
  - Feedback of job performance in every month
  - Freedom to give care to patients
  - Interdepartmental support
  - Sharing of feelings
  - Empowerment
  - Support for learning
- *Sociocultural comfort:*
  - Supportive social environment
  - Participation in making major decisions
  - Information shared by administration
  - Good communication
  - Mentorship
  - Collaboration of nurse-physician
  - Strong leader
- *Environmental comfort:*
  - Strong nursing department
  - Professional environment for practice

- Decreased paper work
- Openness to new ideas.

Pediatric Pain Misconceptions

- Infants and young child do not experience, feel, or remember pain.
- Infants and older children are more sensitive than adults to opioid pain medication.
- Pain is to be endured and can be character-building experiences.
- The risk of opioid addiction prohibits appropriate analgesics.
- Children who are sleeping, playing, or can be distracted are not experiencing pain.

ENHANCING COMFORT FOR CHILDREN

- **Physical comfort:**
  - Homeostasis
  - Medical diagnosis-related issues
  - Pain/comfort management
  - Other physical discomforts
  - Sensory deprivation.
- **Psychospiritual comfort:**
  - Spiritual needs-with parents
  - Anxiety, fear
  - Meaning of illness.
- **Sociocultural comfort:**
  - Fiancé-parents
  - Discharge planning
  - Teaching/information needs
  - Visiting preference-peer groups
  - Continuity of care.
- **Environmental comfort:**
  - Private room
  - Meal preference for family and child
  - Odors, noise, light
  - Play need—age appropriate play materials.

APPLICATIONS

Nursing Education

- Kolcaba's Comfort Theory has significant impacts on the nursing education.

- Students can learn more about the application of Comfort Care Plans on Kolcaba's website.
- Kolcaba's 'Comfort Theory has been included in electronic nursing classification systems such as NANDA (2007–2008), NIC (2001), and NOC (2004)' (Tomey and Alligood, 2010).
- Goodwin, Sener, and Steiner (2007) advocated Kolcaba's concept of holistic comfort as the teaching guideline in the nursing education program.
- Teachers can relieve and ease students' discomforts. Students can transcend into increased motivation, participation, and satisfaction in their lifelong learning.
- To relieve the physical discomfort, teachers encourage students to have good self-care in nutrition and sleep. To provide the psycho-spiritual comfort, teachers give inspiration and positive reassurance to relieve the students' anxieties. To relieve the sociocultural discomfort, teachers show caring and respect for students' different cultural and social backgrounds.
- Goodwin, et al. concluded that teachers and students created an environment with 'a mutually rewarding learning partnership'.

Nursing Practice

- Kolcaba and Wilson (2002) stated that the Theory of Comfort could be applied in perianesthesia nursing.
- Nurses can relieve patients' physical discomfort, such as pain and nausea.
- Patients' psychospiritual comfort needs can be met by comfort measures targeted toward transcendence, such as a massage, mouth care, special visitors, caring touch, and special words of continued encouragement.
- The sociocultural comfort needs can be met by providing 'culturally sensitive reassurance, support... and caring. To provide environmental comfort needs, nurses should try 'to decrease noise, lights, and interrupted sleep to facilitate a peaceful environment'.
- Increased patients' comfort is closely related to patients' positive outcomes for HSBS, such as early ambulation and rehabilitation.
- Health-seeking behaviors are positively related to the improved institutional integrity for the implementation of the best policies and best practices (Kolcaba and Wilson, 2002).

Nursing Research

- Kolcaba's Theory of Comfort is a middle range theory which focusing on comfort as the main concept. Several tools have been created to measure comfort such as the General comfort questionnaire, the visual analog scale, and the Comfort Behaviors Checklist (McEwen and Wills, 2011). Utilizing these instruments, many research studies have been carried out to evaluate Kolcaba's Comfort Theory as it applies to nursing practice and nursing education and to provide direction for future research work.

- Research studies based on theory of comfort have been conducted on many different areas of nursing including 'labor and delivery, peri- and intra-operative care, critical care, burn units, gynecological practice, nursing care of persons with mental or hearing disabilities, emergency air transport, and newborn nurseries' (Kolcaba and DiMarco, 2005).
- Wagner, Byrne, and Kolcaba (2006) uses comfort theory to provide comfort measures to preoperative patients.

LIMITATIONS

- Research studies on the concept of comfort are less and the meaning of comfort has not been defined.
- The concept of comfort might need to be taught to those who do not have skill naturally.
- Comfort theory can mainly use for the nurses' comfort enhancement and improve the practice environments. In reality, the comfort intervention for an adequate nurse staffing is difficult to be achieved.
- The institutions may have the intentions to promote comfort environments based on the theory of comfort but hospital administrators have no enough budget of the organizations.
- Nurses have to take care of many numbers of patients at a time. The increased patient-nurse ratios can increase nurses' discomfort in the work environments.

CRITIQUING THE THEORY

- *Clarity:* She clearly identifies the main components; and easily understandable.
- *Simplicity:* Simple; the theory has few concepts and relationships.
- *Empirical precision:* Comfort theory is used in many research studies has been found testable and applicable in research. This theory provides a theory based on reality.
- *Generality:* It can be used in variety of setting. The comfort theory can be applied to patients of all ages, cultures backgrounds, communities, state or regions. It is also applicable to patients in the hospital, clinic or home. Though it has not necessarily been tested in all of these areas, it can be used to enhance any person's health status in any practice setting.

PRACTICAL APPLICATION OF KOLCABA'S COMFORT THEORY

Example 1: Mrs John, 40-year-old widow underwent hysterectomy. Today is her first postoperative day. She is distress and complaints about the pain in the incision site.

Taxonomic Structure for Ms John's Comfort Needs

	Relief	Ease	Transcedence
Physical	• Incision site pain • immobility	• Restless • Uncomfortable	• He resumes her activities with pain controlled
Psychospritual	• Anxiety • distress	• Visit of relatives • Deep breathing exercises	• Spiritual distress • Questions and doubts
Environment	• Unfamiliar noises • Loud roommate • Lights and temperature	• Lack of privacy • Loss of independence due to immobility	• Need for calm • Need for restfulness
Sociocultural	• Inadequate support from relatives • Financial problem	• Visitors • Phone calls	• She has a supportive network in place, financial issues have been addressed

Comfort Care Actions for Ms John

- *Standard comfort:* Assessment of pain, administration of analgesics, turning or repositioning, frequently check vital signs.
- *Coaching:* Reassurance, emotional support, listening, educate the client, answering questions.
- *Comfort food for the soul:* Diversional therapy, quiet room, calming music, facilitates relatives coming to the bedside, allow periods of undisturbed rest.

Example 2: Master Arun, 10-year-old male child patient, admitted in oncology ward with diagnosis of acute lymphocytic leukemia. He is about to receive his chemotherapy medication when the nurse noticed that the child is alone and crying silently. He is distress and complaints about pain in the incision site.

Comfort Care Actions for Master Arun

- ***Standard comfort:***
  - Assessment for development and complaints of the side effects of the chemotherapy (may use comfort daisies, comfort behavior, checklist, etc.)

	Relief	Ease	Transcedence
Physical	• Mouth sores • Nausea and vomiting • Neuropathy • Diarrhea/ Constipation	Comfortable bed and resting position which facilitates sleep and relaxation	Arun's resumes most of his ADLs with all the side effects controlled
Psychospritual	• Anxiety/fear • Alopecia • Radiation recall	Anticipation of social stigma towards baldness and skin problems	Need for reassurance and support from the healthcare professionals,family and peer group
Environment	Cold room, loud noise and unfamiliar surroundings	Deviation from aseptic technique and standard precaution and Lack of privacy	Need for calm, familiar and positive atmosphere which strictly adheres to infection control guidelines and Need privacy for personal hygienic care
Sociocultural	Absence of family	Failure of effective communication due to language barrier	Need for familial support and reinforcement Need information on his language

- Frequently check vitals and watch out for fever or signs of nosocomial infections.
- Administer medications or treatments to relieve the side effects of chemotherapy.

• ***Coaching:***
  - Avoiding the word 'pain' upon assessment, obtaining data, and rendering health teaching for him.
  - Initiate patient and family education as needed.
• ***Comfort food for the soul:***
  - Practice guided imagery to eliminate factors that could increase physical discomfort.
  - Provide privacy as Marie is entering pubescent stage when she will be concerned about her body image and privacy.

Example 3: Mr Rajesh, 28-year-old male met with a motor vehicle accident and admitted in the trauma department with fracture of left tibia. Apply in Kolcaba Comfort Theory's conceptual framework.

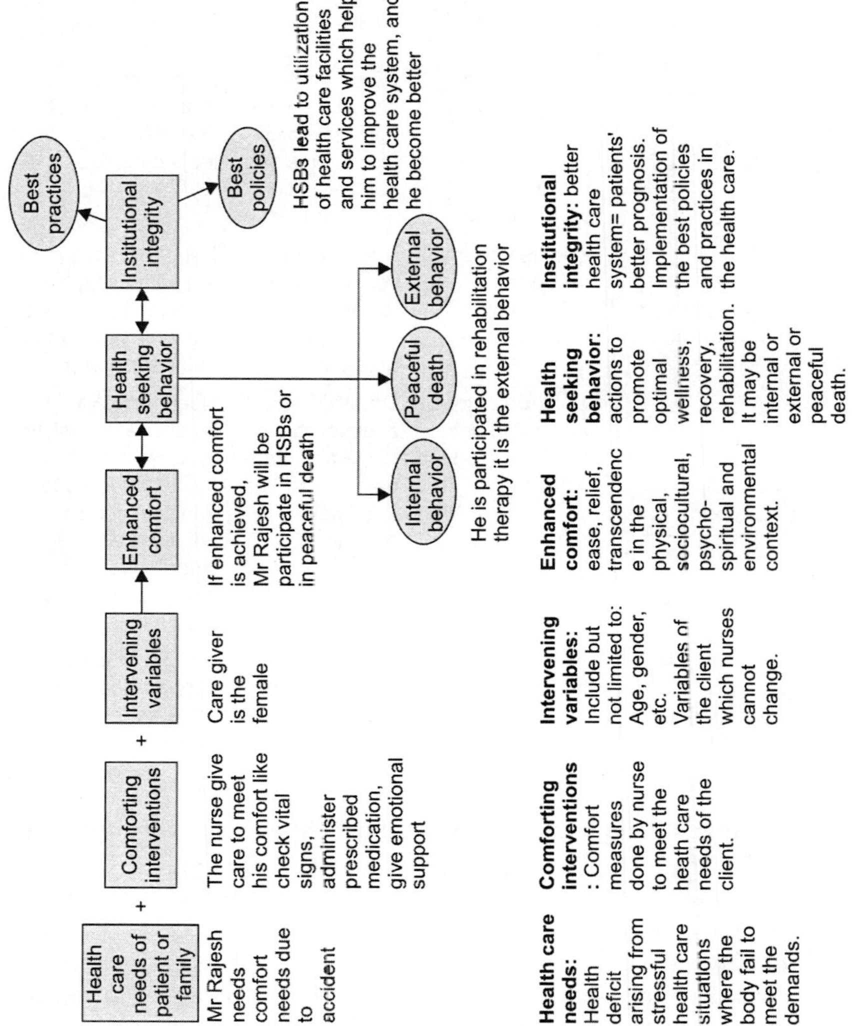

CONCLUSION

There are a lot of benefits one can get in learning and applying Kolcaba's Comfort Theory as it promotes greater understanding and collaboration between health care team members focusing the current shortage in health care team. In addition, this theory will help to improve societal acceptance and appreciation of the health institution and increase patient satisfaction.

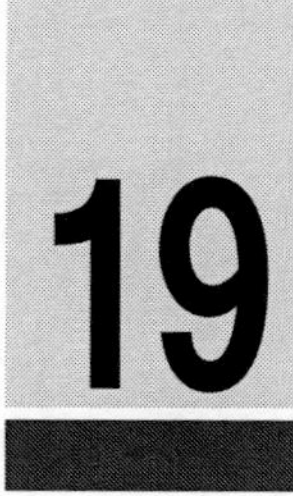

Larrabee J: Quality of Nursing Care

 INTRODUCTION

A theoretical model of quality, based on an organismic worldview, provides a framework for understanding health care quality. This incorporates ethical and economic concepts: value, beneficence, prudence, and justice.

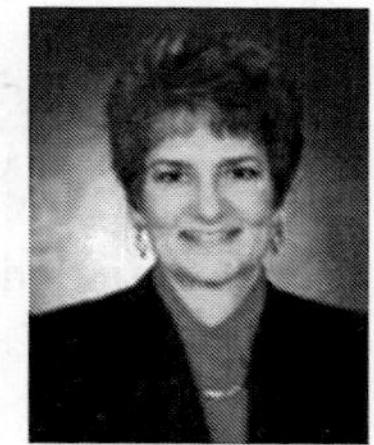

Larrabee J

Biography

- Graduated in Nursing from The Medical College of Georgia.
- Obtained Masters in Nursing from Boston University School of Nursing, and her PhD from The University of Tennessee, Memphis, College of Nursing.
- She worked as a staff nurse, clinical nurse specialist, nursing care quality manager, director of quality improvement, and faculty member.
- She taught at West Virginia University for 13 years.
- Have focused on the quality of health care.

Major Concepts

Quality is defined as 'the presence of socially acceptable, desired attributes within the multifaceted holistic experience of being and doing' and includes four interrelated concepts: value, beneficence, prudence, and justice.

Beneficence is the potentiality or actuality of (a) producing good and (b) promoting well-being' and includes harmlessness. This model proposes that quality and beneficence are interrelated, and empirical evidence supports this relationship.

Values: Something of worth; enduring beliefs or attitudes about the worth of a person, object, idea, or action. They are important because they influence decisions, actions, even nurse's ethical decision-making.

Prudence: A quality in which consistently exhibits good judgment in requesting, reviewing, and weighing information provided by an applicant or recipient, or a person representing an applicant or recipient.

Justice: In which individual people and groups with similar circumstances and conditions should be treated alike; fairness with equal distribution of goods and services.

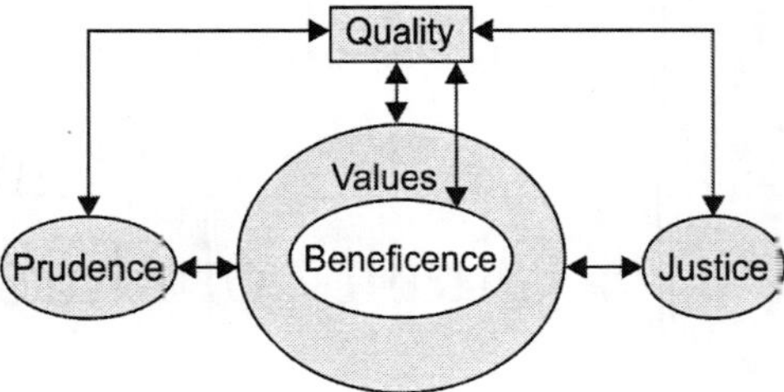

Fig. 19.1: Health care quality model showing concepts and proposed relationship

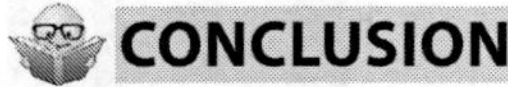

CONCLUSION

The model supports viewing patients and families as equal partners with providers in defining, evaluating, and achieving health care quality.

20

Madeleine M Leininger: Transcultural Nursing

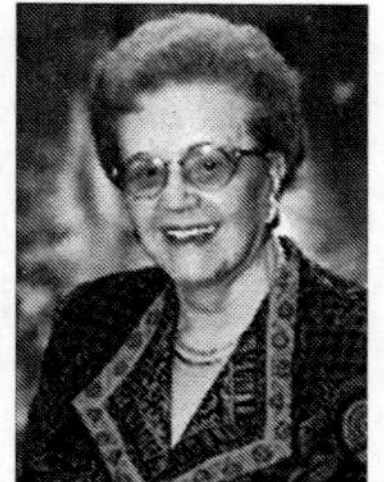

'Essentially transcultural nursing has focused on understanding cultures and their specific care needs and how to provide care that fits their lifeways rather than assuming professional nurses always know what is best for them'.

–Madeleine M Leininger

 INTRODUCTION

Today nurses are facing a world in which they are enforced to use transculturally-based nursing theories and practices in order to care for patients of different cultures. The author Leininger, who in the mid-'50s developed the first transcultural nursing theory with a focus of care of patients, and discusses the relevance, assumptions, and predictions of the culture care theory. She contends that transcultural nursing findings are gradually transforming nursing practice and are providing a new paradigm shift from traditional medical and unicultural practice to multiculturally congruent and specific care modalities.

Biography and Achievements

- She is born in Sutton, Nebraska July 13, 1925.
- She lived on a farm with 4 brothers and sisters.
- She completed her Basic Nursing Education from St. Anthony's School of Nursing, Denver, Colorado in 1948.
- She received her Bachelor of Science from Mount St. Scholastica College (Benedictine College) in Atchison, Kansas in 1950.
- She completed her Master of Science in Psychiatric-Mental Health Nursing from The Catholic University of America in Washington in 1954.
- She received her PhD in Cultural and Social Anthropology from the University of Washington, DC in 1965.
- She is one of the first nursing theorist and transcultural global nursing consultant.
- She developed the concept of transcultural nursing and the ethnonursing research model.
- She is a fellow in the American Academy of Nursing.
- She was named a 'Living Legend' by the American Academy of Nursing in 1998.

- She is a distinguished Fellow of the Royal College of Nursing, Australia.
- She is Professor Emeritus in the College of Nursing, Wayne State University and Adjunct Professor at the University of Nebraska Medical Center, College of Nursing, Omaha.
- Transcultural nursing theory is also known as Culture Care theory.
- Theoretical framework is depicted in her model called the Sunrise Model (1997).

Major Concepts and Definitions

- *Transcultural nursing:* Which means a comparative study of cultures to understand similarities (culture universal) and difference (culture-specific) across human groups.
- *Ethnonursing:* The study of nursing care beliefs, values and practices as cognitively perceived and known by a designated culture through their direct experience, beliefs and value system.
- *Culture:*
  - Set of values, beliefs and traditions, that are held by a specific group of people and handed down from generation to generation.
  - Also beliefs, habits, likes, dislikes, customs and rituals learn from one's family.
  - The learned, shared and transmitted values, beliefs, norms and life way practices of a particular group that guide thinking, decisions, and actions in patterned ways.
  - Culture is learned by each generation through both formal and informal life experiences.
  - Language is primary through means of transmitting culture.
  - The practices of particular culture often arise because of the group's social and physical environment.
  - Culture practice and beliefs are adapted over time but they mainly remain constant as long as they satisfy needs.
- *Religion:* It is a set of belief in a divine or super human power (or powers) to be obeyed and worshipped as the creator and ruler of the universe.
- *Care as a noun:* It is defined as those abstract and concrete phenomena related to assisting, supporting, or enabling experiences or behaviors toward or for others with evident or anticipated needs to ameliorate or improve a human condition or lifeway.
- *Care as a verb:* It is defined as actions and activities directed toward assisting, supporting, or enabling another individual or group with evident or anticipated needs to ameliorate or improve a human condition or lifeway or to face death.
- *Ethnic:* Refers to a group of people who share a common and distinctive culture and who are members of a specific group.
- *Generic (folk or lay) care systems* are culturally learned and transmitted, indigenous (or traditional), folk (home-based) knowledge and skills used to provide assistive, supportive, enabling, or facilitative acts toward or

for another individual, group, or institution with evident or anticipated needs to ameliorate or improve a human life way, health condition (or well-being), or to deal with handicaps and death situations.

- *Emic*: Knowledge gained from direct experience or directly from those who have experienced. It is generic or folk knowledge.
- *Professional care system(s)* are defined as formally taught, learned, and transmitted professional care, health, illness, wellness, and related knowledge and practice skills that prevail in professional institutions usually with multidisciplinary personnel to serve consumers.
- *Professional nursing care (caring)* is defined as formal and cognitively learned professional care knowledge and practice skills obtained through educational institutions that are used to provide assistive, supportive, enabling, or facilitative acts to or for another individual or group in order to improve a human health condition (or well-being), disability, lifeway, or to work with dying clients.
- *Etic:* Knowledge which describes the professional perspective. It is professional care knowledge.
- *Ethnohistory:* Includes those past facts, events, instances, experiences of individuals, groups, cultures, and instructions that are primarily people-centered (ethno) and which describe, explain, and interpret human lifeways within particular cultural contexts and over short or long periods of time.
- *Ethnicity:* A consciousness of belonging to a group.
- *Cultural identity:* The sense of being part of an ethnic group or culture.
- *Culture-universals:* Commonalities of values, norms of behavior, and life patterns that are similar among different cultures.
- *Culture-specifics:* Values, beliefs, and patterns of behavior that tend to be unique to a designate culture.
- *Material culture:* Refers to objects (dress, art, religious artifacts)
- *Non-material culture:* Refers to beliefs customs, languages, social institutions.
- *Subculture:* Composed of people who have a distinct identity but are related to a larger cultural group.
- *Bicultural:* A person who crosses two cultures, lifestyles, and sets of values.
- *Diversity:* Refers to the fact or state of being different. Diversity can occur between cultures and within a cultural group.
- *Acculturation:* People of a minority group tend to assume the attitudes, values, beliefs, find practices of the dominant society resulting in a blended cultural pattern.
- *Cultural shock:* The state of being disoriented or unable to respond to a different cultural environment because of its sudden strangeness, unfamiliarity, and incompatibility to the stranger's perceptions and expectations as it is differentiated from others by symbolic markers (cultures, biology, territory, religion).

- *Cultural imposition* refers to efforts of the outsider, both subtle and not so subtle, to impose his or her own cultural values, beliefs, behaviors upon an individual, family, or group from another culture.
- *Ethnic groups:* Share a common social and cultural heritage that is passed on to successive generations.
- *Ethnic identity:* Refers to a subjective perspective of the person's heritage and to a sense of belonging to a group that is distinguishable from other groups.
- *Race:* The classification of people according to shared biologic characteristics, genetic markers, or features. Not all people of the same race have the same culture.
- *Cultural awareness:* An in-depth self-examination of one's own background, recognizing biases and prejudices and assumptions about other people.
- *Culturally congruent care:* Care that fits the people's valued life patterns and set of meanings—which is generated from the people themselves, rather than based on predetermined criteria.
- *Culturally competent care:* The ability of the practitioner to bridge cultural gaps in caring, work with cultural differences and enable clients and families to achieve meaningful and supportive caring.
- *Worldview* is the way in which people look at the world, or at the universe, and form a 'picture or value stance' about the world and their lives.
- *Cultural and social structure dimensions* are defined as involving the dynamic patterns and features of interrelated structural and organizational factors of a particular culture (subculture or society) which includes religious, kinship (social), political (and legal), economic, educational, technologic and cultural values, ethnohistorical factors, and how these factors may be interrelated and function to influence human behavior in different environmental contexts.
- *Environmental context* is the totality of an event, situation, or particular experience that gives meaning to human expressions, interpretations, and social interactions in particular physical, ecological, sociopolitical and/or cultural settings.
- *Culture care* is defined as the subjectively and objectively learned and transmitted values, beliefs, and patterned lifeways that assist, support, facilitate, or enable another individual or group to maintain their well-being, health, improve their human condition and lifeway, or to deal with illness, handicaps or death.
- *Culture care diversity* indicates the variabilities and/or differences in meanings, patterns, values, lifeways, or symbols of care within or between collectives that are related to assistive, supportive, or enabling human care expressions.
- *Culture care universality* indicates the common, similar, or dominant uniform care meanings, pattern, values, lifeways or symbols that are manifest among many cultures and reflect assistive, supportive, facilitative, or enabling ways to help people.

Nursing Paradigm

- *Human beings:*
  - Humans are believed to be caring and to be capable of being concerned about the needs, well-being and survival of others.
  - Human care is universal, that is, seen in all cultures.
  - Humans are universally caring beings who survive in a diversity of cultures through their ability to provide the universality of care in a variety of ways according to differing cultures, needs and settings.
- *Health:* Defined as a 'state of well-being that is culturally defined, valued and practiced, and which reflects the ability of individuals (or groups) to perform their daily role activities in culturally expressed, beneficial and patterned lifeways.'
- *Environment:*
  - Society or environment are not terms that are defined by Leininger but she instead speaks of worldview, social structure and environmental context.
  - The concept of culture is closely related to society or environment and is considered as a central theme in her theory.
- *Nursing:*
  - Defined as 'a learned humanistic and scientific profession and discipline focused on human care phenomena and caring activities in order to assist, support, facilitate or enable individuals or groups to maintain or regain their health or well-being in culturally meaningful and beneficial ways, or to help individuals face handicaps or death.'
  - Professional nursing care is defined as 'formal and cognitively learned professional care knowledge and practice skills, obtained through educational institutions, that are expected to provide assistive, supportive, enabling or facilitative acts to or for another individual or group in order to improve a human health condition (or well-being), disability, lifeway or to work with dying clients.'
  - Culturally congruent (nursing) care is defined as 'those cognitively based assistive, supportive, facilitative or enabling acts or decisions that are tailor-made to fit with individual, group or institutional cultural values, beliefs and lifeways in order to provide or support meaningful, beneficial and satisfying health care or well-being services.'

Major Assumptions

- Illness and wellness are shaped by various factors including perception and coping skills, as well as the social level of the patient.
- Cultural competence is an important component of nursing.
- Culture influences all spheres of human life. It defines health, illness, and the search for relief from disease or distress.
- Religious and cultural knowledge is an important ingredient in health care.

- The health concepts held by many cultural groups may result in people choosing not to seek modern medical treatment procedures.
- Health care provider need to be flexible in the design of programs, policies, and services to meet the needs and concerns of the culturally diverse population, groups that are likely to be encountered.
- Most cases of lay illness have multiple causalities and may require several different approaches to diagnosis, treatment, and cure including folk and Western medical interventions.
- The use of traditional or alternate models of health care delivery is widely varied and may come into conflict with Western models of health care practice.
- Culture guides behavior into acceptable ways for the people in a specific group as such culture originates and develops within the social structure through interpersonal interactions.
- For a nurse to successfully provide care for a client of a different cultural or ethnic background, effective intercultural communication must take place.

Transcultural Theory Concepts

- Uses culture to understand behavior.
- All cultures are not alike.
- Culture influences all spheres of life. It defines health, illness, and the search for relief from disease or distress.
- Each person viewed as unique with differences that are respected.
- Cultural competence is important in nursing.
- Cultural competence is a combination of culturally congruent behaviors, practice attitudes, and policies that allow nurses to work effectively in cross cultural situations.

The Sunrise Model

Leininger has presented the Sunrise Model to visualize the different dimensions of her Culture Care Theory.

- The concept of culture was derived from anthropology and the concept of care was derived from nursing.
- The ultimate goal of the theory is to provide cultural congruent nursing care practices.
- If one fully discovers care meanings, patterns, and process, one can explain and predict health or well-being.
- Health and care behaviors vary among cultures; therefore nursing care cannot be determined through superficial knowledge and limited contact with a cultural group.
- Nursing care must be based on knowledge by examining social structure, world view, cultural values, language, and environmental contexts.
- This is depicted in the sunrise model.
- Symbolizes the 'rising of the sun (care).

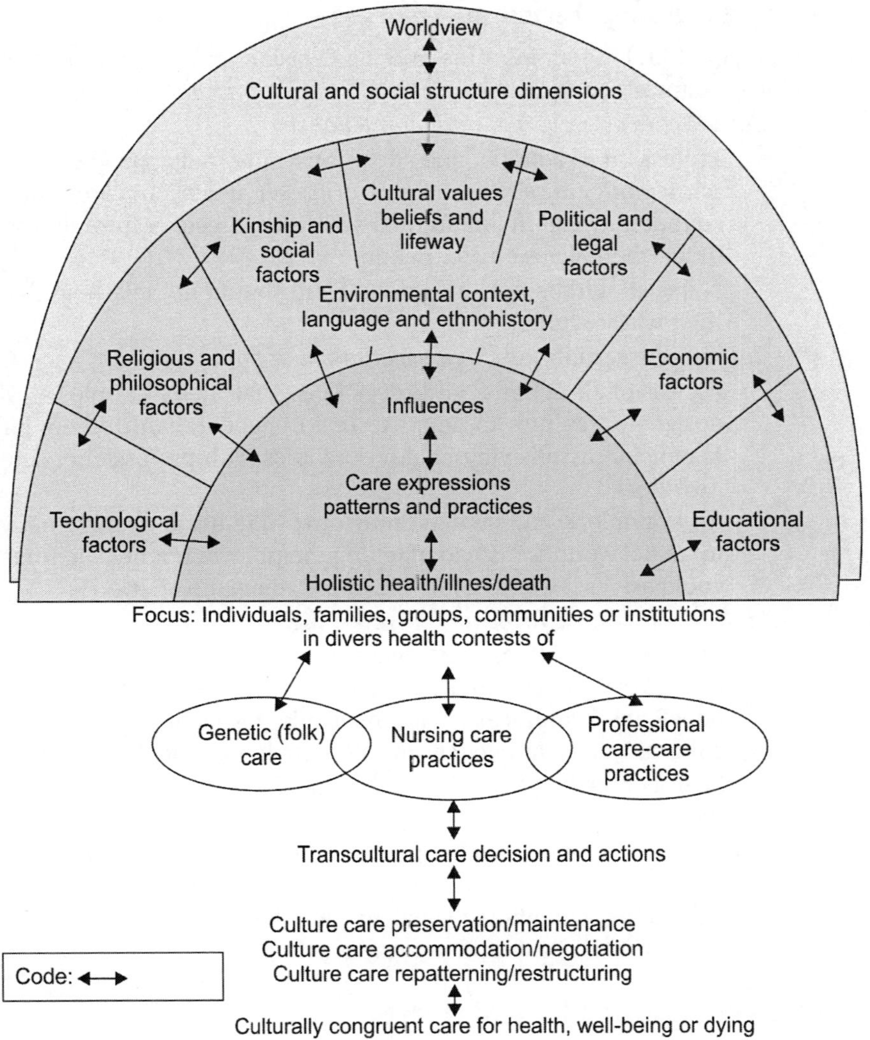

Fig. 20.1: The sunrise model

- The upper half of the circle depicts components of the social structure and world view factors that influence care and health through language and environment. These factors influence the folk, professional, and nursing system(s), which are in the lower half of the model.
- The two halves together form a full sun, which represents the universe that nurses must consider to appreciate human care and health.
- The nursing subsystem can act as a bridge between the folk and personal health systems through the three types of nursing care actions: cultural care preservation, cultural care accommodation, and cultural repatterning.

The Three Nursing Decisions

- Leininger (1991) identified three nursing decision and action modes to achieve culturally congruent care.
  - *Culture care preservation and maintenance:*
    - Professional actions and decisions that help people of a particular culture to retain and/or preserve relevant care values so that they can maintain their well-being, recover from illness, or face handicaps and/or death.
    - Nurse should be non-judgmental and should not tell them that their way is wrong.
  - *Culture care accommodation, negotiation, or both:*
    - Professional actions and decisions that help people of a designated culture to adapt to or to negotiate with others for beneficial or satisfying health outcomes with professional care providers.
    - An example would be if an individual were using a folk remedy to treat a wound. Instead of telling them it will not help, a nurse could ask 'Is it working for you, or are you getting better?'
  - *Culture care restructuring and repatterning:*
    - Professional actions and decisions that help clients reorder, change, or greatly modify their lifeways for new, different, and beneficial health care patterns while respecting the client's cultural values and beliefs and still providing more beneficial or healthier lifeways than before the changes were established with the clients.
    - The nurse could show the patient a different medicine and give them information concerning the new medicine such as it has helped her and others to heal. Explain that it will help if they use it on a regular basis and not just one time.

Nursing Process and Role of Nurse

- The nurse should begin the assessment by attempting to determine the client's cultural heritage and language skills.
- The client should be asked if any of his health beliefs relate to the cause of the illness or to the problem.
- The nurse should then determine what, if any, home remedies the person is taking to treat the symptoms.
- Nurses should evaluate their attitudes toward ethnic nursing care.
- The process of self-evaluation can help the nurse become more comfortable when providing care to clients from diverse backgrounds.
- Nurses have a responsibility to understand the influence of culture, race and ethnicity on the development of social emotional relationship child rearing practices and attitude toward health.
- A child's self-concepts evolves from ideas about his or her social roles.

- Important subculture influences on children include ethnicity social class, occupation school peers and mass culture.
- Socioeconomic influences play major role in ability to seek opportunity for health promotion for wellness.
- Religious practices greatly influence health promotion belief in families.
- Many ethnic and cultural groups in country retain the cultural heritage of their original culture.
- How culture influences behaviors, attitudes, and values depends on many factors and thus is not the same for different members of a cultural group.
- The nurse should have an understanding of the general characteristics of the major ethnic groups, but should always individualize care rather than generalize about all clients in these groups.
- Before assessing the cultural background of a client, nurses should assess how they are influenced by their own culture.
- The nursing diagnosis for clients should include potential problems in their interaction with the health care system and problems involving the effects of culture.
- The planning and implementation of nursing interventions should be adapted as much as possible to the client's cultural background.
- Evaluation should include the nurse's self-evaluation of attitudes and emotions toward providing nursing care to clients from diverse sociocultural backgrounds.
- The client's educational level and language skills should be considered when planning teaching activities.
- Discussing cultural questions related to care with the client and family during the planning stage helps the nurse understand how cultural variables are related to the client's health beliefs and practices, so that interventions can be individualized for the client.
- Evaluation continues throughout the nursing process and should include feedback from the client and family.
- Self-evaluation by the nurse is crucial as he or she increases skills for interaction.

Limitations

- It can also be the primary cause of error in making clinical decisions like misperception of the outcomes and misperception of the values patients place on to outcomes. Not all the data that will be taken will be accurate and applicable to all clients. We should also consider the uniqueness of individual.
- If nursing practices fail to recognize culturological aspects of human needs, there will be signs of less efficacious nursing care practices and dissatisfaction with nursing services (Leininger). Does it mean that a sole principle in providing efficient care is the culturally consistent care? It can be an aspect but it does not mean that we will not consider the other

important things, because we need to remember that we should also provide holistic care, not only in the concept of culture.
- This theory does not give any attention to the disease, symptoms, etc.
- There can be a problem in adapting or integrating the culture of the other which can be the cause of cultural shock on the part of the nurses. Studying culture does not mean that we could already relate to them, studying is different from actual experience.
- The limited applicability of a static culture framework, lack of attention to the structural context in which health care issues arise and must be addressed, and the consequent inappropriateness of many health care strategies based on cultural framework.

Application

- *Nursing practice:*
  - Accepted in the nursing practice.
  - Communities are becoming more multicultural, and health personnel are being expected to respond to client's diverse cultural needs. Immigrants and people from unfamiliar cultures are generally expecting nurses to respect their cultural values, beliefs, and lifeways.
- *Nursing education:* Since 1980, an increasing number of nursing curricula emphasize transcultural nursing and care.
- *Nursing research:* Several research nurses are testing transcultural nursing in US and other countries. Many cultures have been studied utilizing this theory.

Critique

- *Simplicity:* Not simple; truly transcultural, global in scope, and highly complex; holistic and comprehensive.
- *Generality:* General; qualitatively-oriented theory that is broad, comprehensive, and worldwide in scope; useful and applicable to groups and individuals with the goal of rendering culture-specific nursing care.
- *Empirical precision:* Researchable; qualitative research has been the primary paradigm to discover largely unknown phenomena of care and health in diverse cultures.
- *Derivable consequences:* It has important outcomes for nursing; culture-specific care is necessary and essential new goal in nursing; useful and applicable to nursing practice, education, and research.

PRACTICAL APPLICATION OF LEININGER'S CULTURAL CARE THEORY

Mr Ankit is 55-year-old naïve Asian who is member of tribe community. Mr Ankit is overweight and has come to the clinic with his wife, who is also overweight. He complaints of symptoms congruent with elevated blood pressure.

The nurse at the clinic is not a member of Mr Ankit's culture but has worked in this clinic which serves a medical home for the local tribe community for many years. In the past, she has participated in the culture (albeit as an outsider), observed of cultural group, and interviewed members of the cultural group. Thus is familiar with the worldview of the members of the culture, although she acknowledges that the worldviews of different generations within the tribe group tend to differ somewhat. In general, she knows the lifeways, cultural values, and environmental context of this particular cultural group. She is also familiar with patterns within the tribe group, many of whom suffer disease associated with being overweight such as hypertension and diabetes. Specifically, the nurse recognizes that this problem is associated with a diet and sedentary lifestyle that are incongruent with the historical lifeways of Asian culture. Assessment that collected during her interview with Mr Ankit reveal that lifestyle is sedentary and that he eats a diet high in saturated fat. Mr Ankit's BP is also a range that is slightly higher than normal.

The Sunrise Enabler will be useful tool for the nurse as she continues to systematically explore the components of the patient's culture during the process of planning care. During the planning phase, the nurse develops a plan of care based on the data gathered and presents the plan to Mr. Ankit and his wife for review and modifications. This process should result in culture care preservation or maintenance, accommodation, and repatterning because the nurse implements the plan to promote health and well-being of Mr. Ankit and his family in a way that is both congruent with the lifeways of tribe community and congruent with current best practices. Evaluation is based on the nurse's observation that the process has resulted in culturally congruent nursing care for Mr Ankit and his family.

Throughout this process, the model may be applied simultaneously to other problems as they are identified by Mr Ankit and the nurse. Culturally congruent strategies will be planned to address those issues that are compatible with current clinical practices.

CONCLUSION

It remains one of the oldest, most holistic, and most comprehensive theories to generate knowledge of diverse and similar cultures worldwide. The theory has been a powerful means to discover largely unknown knowledge in nursing and the health fields. It provides a new mode to assure culturally competent, safe, and congruent transcultural nursing care.

21 Rozzano Locsin: Technological Competency

INTRODUCTION

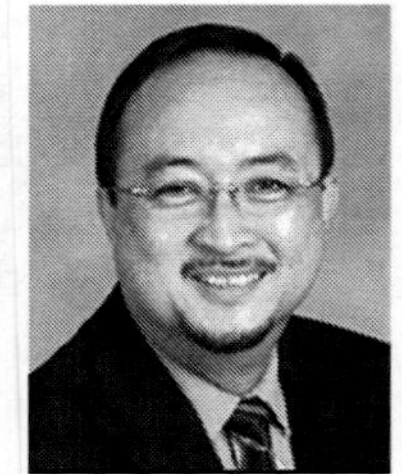

Rozzano Locsin

Rozzano Locsin developed this theory since shifting of nursing profession towards, technology. Technological competency in nursing fosters the recognition and realization of persons as participants in their care rather than as objects of care.

Biography

- Graduated in Nursing from Silliman University, Philippines in 1976.
- He received Masters degree in Nursing from Silliman University, Philippines in 1978.
- He conferred Doctorate in Nursing from University of the Philippines, Manila, Philippines in 1988.
- His research areas are mainly in technology and caring in nursing.

Assumptions

- Persons are whole or complete in the moment.
- Knowing persons is a practice process of nursing that allows for continuous appreciation of person moment to moment.
- Nursing is a discipline and professional practice.
- Technology is used to know persons fully in the moment.

Major Concepts

Dimensions of Technological Value in the Theory

- Technology as completing human beings to re-formulate the ideal human being, such as in replacement parts, both mechanical (prostheses) or organic (transplantation of organs).
- Technology as machine technologies, e.g. computers and gadgets enhancing nursing activities to provide quality patient care.
- Technologies that mimic human beings and human activities to meet the demands of nursing care practices.

Technological Competency as Caring in Nursing

- Technological competency as caring in nursing is the harmonious coexistence between technologies and caring in nursing.
- The harmonization of these concepts places the practice of nursing within the context of modern healthcare and acknowledges that these concepts can co-exist.
- Technology brings the patient closer to the nurse. Conversely, technology can also increase the gap between the nurse and nursed.
- When technology is used to know persons continuously in the moment, the process of nursing is lived.

Nursing Process

a. *Knowing:* The process of knowing person is guided by technological knowing in which persons are appreciated as participants in their care rather than as objects of care. The nurse enters the world of the other. In this process, technology is used to magnify the aspect of the person that requires revealing—a representation of the real person.

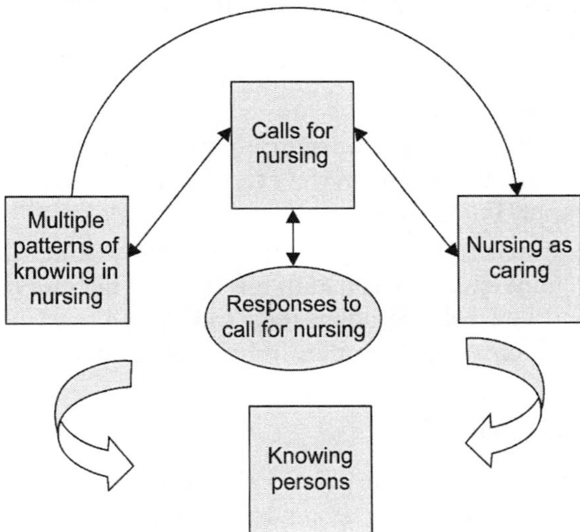

Fig. 21.1: Framework for knowing the person

b. *Designing:* Both the nurse and the one nursed plan a mutual care process from which the nurse can organize a rewarding nursing practice, i.e. responsive to the patient's desire for care.

c. *Participation in appreciation:* The simultaneous practice of conjoined activities which are crucial to knowing persons. In this stage of the process is the alternating rhythm of implementation and evaluation. The evidence of continuous knowing, implementation and participation is reflective of the cyclical process of knowing persons.

d. *Verifying knowledge:* The continuous, circular process demonstrates the ever-changing, dynamic nature of knowing in nursing. Knowledge about the person, i.e. derived from knowing, designing, and implementing further informs the nurse and the one.

Metaparadigam in Nursing

Person: This includes both individuals and human groups. A 'whole' person, complete in the moment and continually growing, changing in response to unique personal conditions, and experiences.

Health: It is the 'enhancing of personhood,' allowing each person to develop and progress moment to moment.

Environment: Human beings' physical surroundings, the significant individuals and groups in their lives, and their social, political and economic context as they are associated to health and well-being.

Nursing: The concepts of caring and intentionality, compassion, confidence, commitment and conscience are all essential components of caring in nursing.

Critique of Technological Competency Caring in Nursing

Clarity: Though all the concepts in this theory is consistent, it is observed that meaning of these concepts are bit confusing.

Simplicity: This theory is very simple, but when technological nursing competence is complex in nature.

Generality: Though this theory started to apply in the intensive care units, due to technological advancements in the every area of health care system this theory can be apply into all fields.

Derivable consequences: With advancements in these and other aspects of health care technology, such as health information technology, nurses will continue to find new ways to adapt their care as patients seek health and wholeness in an increasingly complex technological environment.

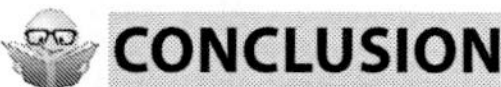

CONCLUSION

As nursing heads in the direction of becoming more technology-focused, this theory will only become more relevant. In the current climate of nursing it is all too important for a nurse to competent in the use of technology.

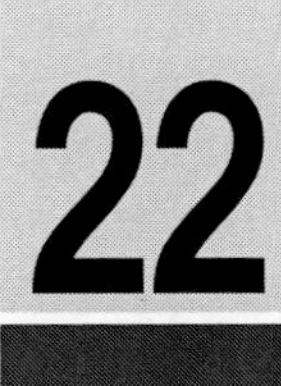

Ida Jean Orlando: The Deliberative Nursing Process

'Patients have their own meanings and interpretations of situations and therefore nurses must validate their inferences and analyses with patients before drawing conclusions.'

–Ida Jean Orlando

INTRODUCTION

Nurse communicates with the patient and tries to plan care for the patient daily. But unexpected troubles to the patient's recovery may arise at any time; this can affect the planned care. At this time, nurse should aware how to deal with those problems and which help patient to regain his or her well-being. Ida Jean Orlando developed *Deliberative Nursing Process* that help nurses to prepare an effective nursing care plan and this can also be easily adapted when and if any complexity come up with the patient at any time.

Biography

- Ida Jean Orlando, a first-generation American of Italian descent was born on August 12, in 1926.
- She felt that nursing was an opportunity for her to grow beyond her family boundaries.
- She is married to Robert Pelletier and lives in the Boston area.
- She passed away on November 28, 2007.

Achievements

- She received diploma in nursing from New York Medical College, Flower Avenue Hospital School of Nursing in New York in the year 1947.
- In 1951, she received a BS in public Health Nursing from St. Johns University in Brooklyn.
- In 1954, she completed her MA in Mental health consultation from Columbia University teachers College, New York.
- Orlando was an Associate Professor at Yale School of Nursing where she was Director of the Graduate Program in Mental Health Psychiatric Nursing.
- She was project investigator of a National Institute of Mental Health (NIMH) grant entitled at Yale: Integration of Mental Health Concepts in a Basic Nursing Curriculum Research.

- It was from her research Integration of Mental Health Concepts in a Basic Nursing Curriculum Research; Orlando developed her theory which was published in her 1961 book. *The Dynamic Nurse-Patient Relationship* and revised 1972 book.
- She furthered the development of her theory when at McLean Hospital in Belmont, MA as Director of a Research Project: Two Systems of Nursing in a Psychiatric Hospital. The results of this research are contained in her 1972 book titled: *The Discipline and Teaching of Nursing Process.*
- Orlando held various positions in the Boston area, and she was a board member of Harvard Community Health Plan.
- She served as both a national and international consultant.
- She served as a frequent lecturer and conducted numerous seminars on nursing process.

CONCEPTS OF ORLANDO

She describes her model as a revolving around five major interrelated concepts they are the following:

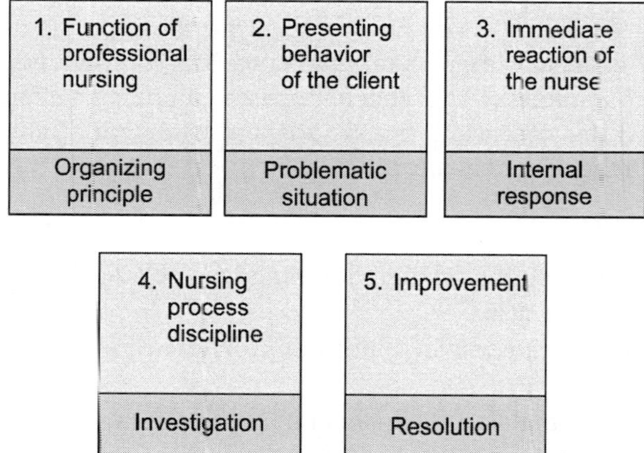

Fig. 22.1: Framework for deliberative nursing process

- **Functions of a professional nursing**
  - The function of professional nursing is the organizing principle.
  - This means finding out and meeting the patient's immediate needs for help.
  - According to Orlando, 'Nursing is responsive to individuals who suffer or anticipate a sense of helplessness, it is focused on the process of care in an immediate experience, and it is concerned with providing direct assistance to individuals in whatever setting they are found for the purpose of avoiding, relieving, diminishing or curing the individual's sense of helplessness.'

- The function of nursing to help the patient to meet his needs. That is, if the patient has an immediate need for help, and the nurse discovers and meets that need, the purpose of nursing has been achieved.

- **Presenting behavior of the client**
  - Problematic situation of the patient is the presenting behavior.
  - Through the presenting behavior of the client, the nurse recognizes the patient's immediate need for help. To find out the immediate need for help the nurse must first distinguish the situation as problematic.
  - According to Orlando, 'presenting behavior of the patient, regardless of the from in which it appears, may present plea for help.'
  - The presenting behavior of the client, which is the stimulus, causes an automatic internal response in the nurse, which in turn causes a response in the client.
  - Patient behavior may be *verbal* or *nonverbal* which alerts the nurse that the patient needs help.
- **Immediate reaction of the nurse**
  - Immediate reaction of the nurse is the internal response.
  - Nurse's reaction is comprised of three sequential parts (Orlando, 1972). First, the nurse perceives the behavior with her five senses. Second, this perception leads to automatic thought in the nurse. Finally, the thought produces an automatic feeling, causing the person to act. These three items are the patient's immediate response.
  - The immediate response reflects how the nurse experiences her participation in the nurse-client relationship. The beginning of the nurse-patient relationship takes place in this part.
  - In 1972, Orlando depicts a diagram showing open sharing of nurse' reaction *vs* keeping the reaction s secret. Only openness in sharing the nurse's reaction assures that client's need will be successfully resolved.

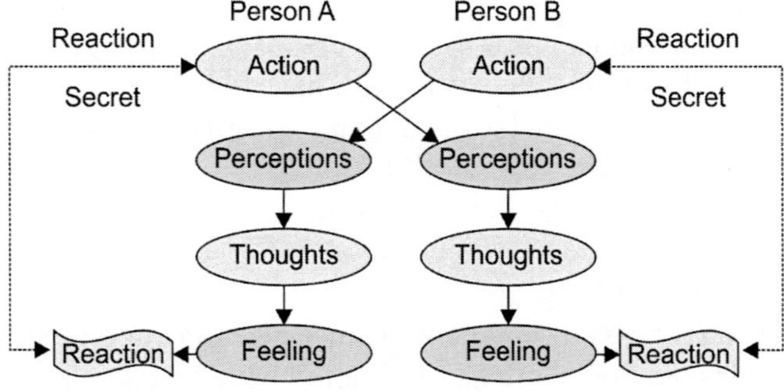

Fig. 22.2: Secret reaction of the nurse

The action process in a person-to-person contact functioning by open disclosure. The perceptions, thoughts, and feelings of each individual are directly available to the perception of the other individual through the observable action.

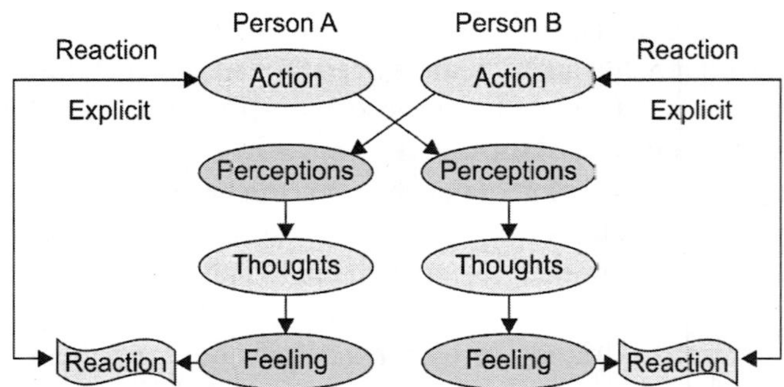

Fig. 22.3: Explicit reaction of the nurse

The action process in a person-to-person contact functioning in secret. The perceptions, thoughts, and feelings of each individual are not directly available to the perception of the other individual through the observable action.

Nurse's Action

- In 1990, Orlando includes 'only what she [the nurse] says or does with or for the benefit of the patient' as professional nursing action. 'The nurse initiates a process of exploration to ascertain how the patient is affected by what she says or does.'
- The nurse can act in two ways: Automatic or deliberative. Only the second manner fulfills her professional function.
- **Automatic actions** are 'those decided upon for reasons other than the patient's immediate need,' whereas **deliberative actions** ascertain and meet this need.
- The following are the criteria for deliberative actions:
  - The correct identification of patient needs by validation of the nurse's reaction to the patient behavior results deliberative actions.
  - The nurse explores the meaning of the action with the patient and its significance to meeting his need.
  - The nurse validates the action's effectiveness immediately after completing it.
  - The nurse is free of stimuli unrelated to the patient's need when she acts.

- **Nursing process discipline**
  - Nursing process discipline is the investigation into the client's need.
  - Any observation shared and explored with the client is immediately useful in ascertaining and meeting his need, or finding out he has no needs at that time.
  - The nurse cannot think that any aspect of her reaction to the client is correct, helpful, or appropriate until she checks the validity of it. Exploration with the patient helps validate the patient's behavior.

- The nurse initiates this exploration to find out how the client is affected by what he or she says and does.
- Automatic reactions are ineffective because the nurse's action is determined for reasons other than the meaning of the patient's behavior or the patient's immediate need for help.
- When the nurse does not explore the patient's reaction with him, it is reasonably certain that effective communication between nurse and patient stops.

- **Improvement**
  - Improvement is the resolution to the patient's situation.
  - The nurse decides on a suitable action to resolve the need in cooperation with the patient.
  - In the resolution, the nurse's actions are not evaluated. Instead, the result of her actions is evaluated to determine whether her actions served to help the client communicate his need for help and how it was met. If the client behavior improves, the action was successful and the process is completed. If there is no change or the behavior gets worse, the process recycles with new efforts to clarify the client's behavior or the appropriate nursing action.
  - In each contact, the nurse repeats a process of learning which can help the patient.
  - The nurse's own individuality, as well as that of the client, requires going through this each time the nurse is called upon to render service to those who need her.

PARADIGM OF ORLANDO'S THEORY

Orlando includes human, health, and nursing. But not included environment.

- **Human being:**
  - Orlando uses the concept of human as she emphasizes individuality and the dynamic nature of the nurse-patient relationship.
  - She assumes person behave verbally or nonverbally relationship.
  - For her, human in need are the focus of nursing practice.
- **Health:**
  - Orlando does not define health, it is implied.
  - Assumes freedom from mental or physical discomfort, feelings of adequacy and well-being contribute to health.
  - The concept of health replaces helplessness as the initiator of a necessity for nursing. Orlando stated that nursing deals with human beings who are in need of help.
- **Nursing:**
  - Orlando assumes, nursing as unique and independent in its concerns for an individual's need for help in an immediate situation.
  - The efforts to meet the individual's need for help are carried out in an interactive situation and in a disciplined manner that requires proper training.

ASSUMPTIONS

Orlando's model of nursing makes the following assumptions:

- When clients are not capable to cope with their needs on their own, they become distressed by feelings of helplessness.
- In its professional character, nursing adds to the distress of the patient.
- Patients are unique and individual in their responds.
- Nursing offers mothering and nursing analogous to an adult who mothers and nurtures a child.
- Nursing deals with people, environment, and health.
- Patients need help communicating their needs; they are not comfortable and ambivalent about their dependency needs.
- Individuals are able to be secretive or explicit about their needs, perceptions, thoughts, and feelings.
- The nurse-patient situation is dynamic; actions and reactions are influenced by both the nurse and the patient.
- Individual attach meanings to situations and actions that are not apparent to others.
- Nurse is concerned with needs that clients cannot meet on their own needs independently.
- Clients enter into nursing care through medicine.
- The client is unable to state the nature and meaning of his distress without the help of the nurse, or without her first having established a helpful relationship with the patient.
- Any observation shared and observed with the patient is immediately helpful in ascertaining and meeting his need, or finding out that he is not in need at that time.

Characteristics of the Theory

- Orlando's theory provides a reasonable and sequential process for nursing.
- Orlando's theory interrelate concepts.
- Orlando's theory has a logical nature.
- Orlando's theory is simple and applicable in the daily practice.
- Orlando's theory does not conflict with other validated theories.
- Orlando's theory contributes to the professional knowledge.
- Orlando's theory is applicable in all nursing practice.

NURSING PROCESS

Orlando's nursing process discipline can be compared with the present nursing process. Certain over all characteristics are similar in both processes. Both nursing processes need interpersonal relationship, i.e. interaction between nurse and patient which requires effective communication techniques.

The Deliberative Nursing Process has five stages: Assessment, diagnosis, planning, implementation, and evaluation.

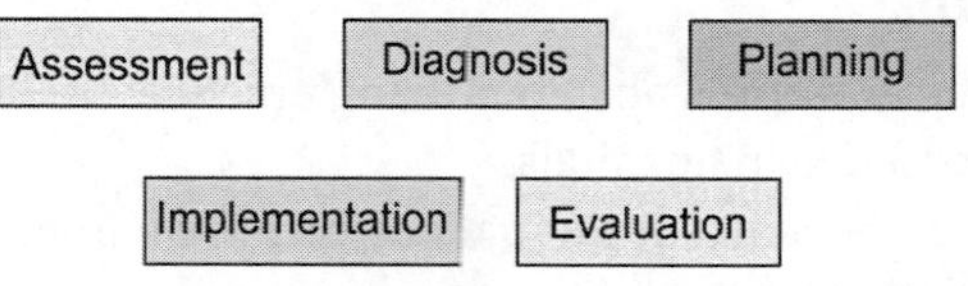

Fig. 22.4: Deliberative nursing process

- **Assessment**
  - This phase of nursing process means sharing of **nurse's reaction** to the patient's behavior. This means patient behavior help to start the assessment.
  - Assessment is done from direct or indirect data. Direct data means any perception; thought or feeling the nurse has from her own experience of the patient's behavior at any or several moments in time. Indirect data means records of other health members.
  - In the assessment stage, the nurse completes a holistic assessment of the patient's needs.
- **Nursing Diagnosis**
  - The nurse makes clinical judgment about health problems in the diagnosis stage.
  - The diagnosis can then be confirmed using links to defining characteristics, related factors, and risk factors found in the patient's assessment.
  - Exploration of the nurse's reaction with the patient in the Orlando's process leads to identification of his **need for help**.
- **Planning**
  - The planning phase addresses each of the problems identified in the diagnosis.
  - Each problem is given a specific goal or outcome, and each goal or outcome is given nursing interventions to help achieve the goal.
  - By the end of this stage, the nurse will have a nursing care plan.
  - This stage corresponds to the **nurse's action** phase of the Orlando's process.
- **Implementation**
  - The nurse begins using the nursing care plan, in the implementation stage.
  - It involves the final selection and carrying out of the planned action.
  - This is also the part of **nurse's action** phase of the Orlando's process.
- **Evaluation**
  - Finally, in the evaluation stage, the nurse looks at the improvement of the patient toward the goals set in the nursing care plan.
  - Changes can be made to the nursing care plan based on how well the patient is improving towards the goals. If any new problems are identified in the evaluation stage, they can be reassessed.
  - It is also the part of **nurse's action** phase of the Orlando's process.

APPLICATIONS

Nursing Practice

- Orlando's theory is applicable to nursing practice.
- It is basis of practice in hospitals.
- This theory can be used at the patient care level, managerial level, and nursing division level.
- Brighton Gardens Assisted Living, Cherry Hill, New Jersey, USA (2002) uses Orlando's deliberative nursing process theory: A practice application in an extended care facility.

Nursing Education

- Orlando's process has made a considerable contribution to nursing education.
- Samereh Abdoli, PhD and Shadi Satat Safavi, MSc (2010) uses Orlando's theory in nursing students' immediate responses to distressed clients.

Nursing Research

- Enjoyed considerable acceptance by the nursing profession in the area of research.
- This theory has been applied to a variety of research settings in nursing field.
- RI Shea, McBride, Gavin, and Bauer (198), in a Veterans Administration (VA) ambulatory psychiatric practice in Providence, used Orlando's theoretical model with patients having a bipolar disorder.

Limitations

- The theory lacks the concept of environment which limits the development of research hypothesis.
- The theory not focuses on long-term care because the theory mainly focused on immediate situation.

Critiquing the Theory

- *Clarity:* Clear; involves defining concepts simply at first and then developing them throughout her books.
- *Simplicity:* The theory has few concepts and relationships.
- *Empirical precision:* Orlando's theory is used in many research work has been found testable and applicable in research.
- *Generality:* Focuses on a limited number of situations; it could be modified and can be used in other nursing situations and other professional fields.

PRACTICAL APPLICATION OF ORLANDO NURSING PROCESS

Mr Raj, 21 years old BTECH student undergone appendectomy. Today is his first postoperative day. His preference for room temperature not more than 20 °C and he is resting comfortably with this temperature. A patient, 85-year-old man has shifted to Mr Raj's room after his surgery that has loudly and frequently complained that the room is too cold. The nurse just entered the room and seems that Mr Raj is restless.

Patient behavior	Nurse's reaction	Nurse's action
• Mr Raj is moving restlessy in his bed. • Previously, he was sleeping.	• The nurse perceive that Mr Raj is now restless, feel that he may be in pain. • The nurse asks him that whether he need analgesic. • He answers that he is not in pain and he just want to sleep. • At this moment the roomate loudly complaint about room is too cold. • Then nurse perceive the reason for his restlessness and ask him, he said yes. • Thus the nurse validate her perception.	• The nurse arrange another roomate closer to his age. • Within 30 minutes of taking this deliberative action, nurse note that he is once again resting quietly, thus validating that the action was effective.

CONCLUSION

Orlando was one of the first nursing leaders to identify and emphasize the elements of nursing process. Orlando's theory mainly focus on the function of nursing. The theory provides a framework for nursing, but the use of her theory does not exclude nurses from using other nursing theories while caring for patients.

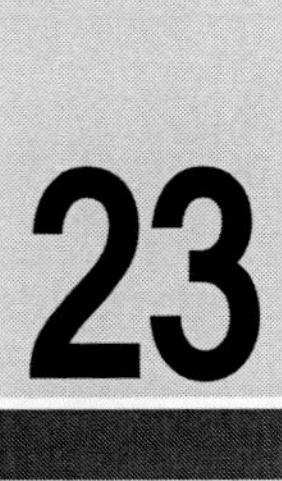

Rosenstock, Strecher and Becker: Health Belief Model

 INTRODUCTION

In nursing profession Health Belief Model (HBM) is popular, mainly in issues focusing on patient compliance and preventive health care practices. Health Belief Model provide a way of understanding and predicting how clients will behave in relation to their health and how will comply with health care therapies. This model depicts the relationship between a person's belief and behavior. Health Belief Model is one of the most popular and widely used theories in intervention science.

History

- The HBM is a cognitive-behavioral model that explains and predicts health behaviors. This is done by focusing on the attitudes and beliefs of individuals.
- The HBM was first developed in the 1950s by a group of social psychologists Godfrey Hochbaum, Stephen Kegels, Irwin Rosenstock working in the US Public Health Services.
- The model was developed in response to explain why people were not participating in disease detection programs (Tuberculosis Screening). Since then, the HBM has been adapted to explore a variety of long- and short-term health behaviors, including sexual risk behaviors and the transmission of HIV/AIDS.
- Firstly HBM developed to predict preventive health behavior, revised to include general health motivation.
- Only four key concepts: *Perceived susceptibility, perceived severity, perceived benefits, and perceived barriers* were first presented in the model.
- Later to 'stimulate behavior' the concept of *Cues for Action* was added.
- Finally, in 1988, the concept of *self-efficacy* was added to address the challenges of habitual unhealthy behaviors, such as smoking and overeating by Irwin M Rosenstock, Victor J Strecher, and Marshall H Becker. The model has been revised to apply to a greater number of people (Expanded).
- The HBM is derived to a great extent from the theories of psychologist Kurt Lewin, who suggested that people exit in a life space, composed of regions of with positive and negative values.

Assumptions of HBM

An individual will take health-related action if that individual:

- Feels that a negative health condition can be avoided.
- Has a positive belief that taking a recommended actions helps to avoid a negative health condition.
- Expects that he/she can effectively take a recommended action confidently.

Components and Concepts of Health Belief Model

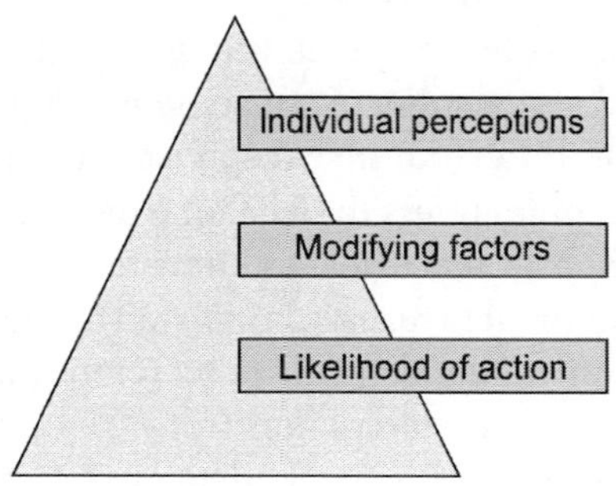

Fig. 23.1: Components of health belief model

- **Individual perceptions:** Individual perceptions is based on three perceptions.
  - ***Perceived susceptibility to a disease:***
    - An individual's perception that chance of getting the disease. People can vary greatly in regards to their perception of susceptibility.
    - On one extreme are individuals who completely deny any possibility of acquiring the disease.
    - In the middle are people who admit to the possibility of acquiring disease, but believe it will not likely happen to them.
    - At the other end are people who are so fearful of acquiring the disease that they believe that they will in all probability acquire it.
    - The more susceptible a person feels, the greater the likelihood they will take preventive measures.
      Examples: Use of condoms to decrease the susceptibility to HIV infection, use of sunscreen to prevent skin cancer screen.
  - **Perceived seriousness of a disease:**
    - An individual's belief about the seriousness or severity of a disease. People vary on their level of perceive severity also.
    - One might only be concerned with the medical perspective and worry about the signs, symptoms, and disabilities caused by the disease. They also are concerned temporary or permanent nature of the condition and its potential for death.

    - Another individual might look at the disease from a broader perspective, such as acquiring the disease would affect their family, their job, and their relationships.
      For example: Flu is a minor ailment. It will subside if one takes rest in home. If one has asthma, contracting with flu will admit in hospital. In this case ones perception of the flu might be that it is a serious disease. Another example is that if one is self-employed, having flu might mean a week or more lost wages. So this would influence one's perception of the seriousness of that disease.
  - **Perceived threat of a disease:**
    - The combination of perceived susceptibility to a disease and perceived seriousness of a disease is the perceived threat of the health condition (emotive response is fear).
    - This perception refers to belief of a person about whether or not a disease poses real threat to him/her.
    - Perceived threat to disease is affected by modifying factors. These factors can influence both perception and the corresponding cues necessary to start action.
      For example: The perceived threat of a heart attack can be used to motivate a person with high blood pressure to do exercise daily.
- **Modifying factors:** Factors that modify person's perception.
  - ***Demographic variables:***
    - It includes age, sex, race, and ethnicity.
      For example: An infant does not perceive the importance of a healthy diet. An adolescent may perceive peer approval as more important than family approval and may participate in hazardous activities or adopt unhealthy eating and sleeping patterns.
  - ***Sociopsychological variables:***
    - Personality, social class, influence from peers or other reference group pressure (e.g. self-help or vocational group) may encourage preventive health behaviors even when individual motivation is low.
    - Expectations of others may motivate people:
      For example: Not to drive car after drinking alcohol.
  - **Structural variables:**
    - Knowledge about the disease and prior contact with the disease are the structural variables that are prescribed to influence preventive behavior.
      For example: Higher adherence rates with prescribed treatment among mothers whose children had frequent fever and diarrhea.
  - **Cues to action:**
    - It may be internal or external.
    - *Internal cues*: Include fatigue, uncomplicated symptoms, or thought about the condition of an illness who is close.

- *External cues*: Includes mass media campaigns, advice from others, reminder post card form, physician or dentist, illness of family member or friend, and newspaper or magazine article.
- Cues to action need to be strong enough to include the person who believes that he has low susceptibility to an illness, if they are to be successful.

  For example: Women attend breast cancer education program when he came to know that his friend is suffering from breast cancer.

- **Likelihood of action:** Likelihood of a person's taking preventive health action depends on the perceived benefits of the action minus perceived barriers to action.
  - ***Perceived benefits of preventive action:***
    - This refers to a person's perception of the effectiveness of various actions available to reduce the threat of illness or disease or to cure disease.
    - The course of action a person takes in preventing or curing disease relies on consideration and evaluation of both perceived susceptibility and perceived benefit, such that the person would accept the recommended health action if it was perceived as beneficial.
    - Perceived benefits of preventive action help whether a new behavior is better than what he is already doing.

      For example: Refraining from smoking to prevent lung cancer, eating nutritious foods and avoiding junk foods to maintain weight.
  - **Perceived barriers to preventive action:**
    - It refers to a one's feelings on the obstacles to performing a recommended health action.
    - There is large variation in a person's feelings of barriers, or impediments, which lead to a cost/benefit analysis.
    - The person weighs the effectiveness of the actions against the perceptions that it may be expensive, dangerous (e.g. side effects), unpleasant (e.g. painful), time-consuming, or inconvenient, life style changes.

      For example: Women's not doing Pap smear test to detect cervical cancer, due to fear that the test is painful.
  - **Likelihood of taking recommended preventive health action:**
    - The individual take preventive health action based on his perception of the benefit of taking action.

      For example: Life-style changes, increased adherence to medical treatment, seek for medical advice or treatment.
  - **Self efficacy:**
    - This component is added later on (in 1988 by Rosenstock, Strecher and Beckers).
    - It means confidence in a person's ability to adopt a behavior.

For example: Provide training, guidance in performing action, confident doing BSE in order to prevent breast cancer.

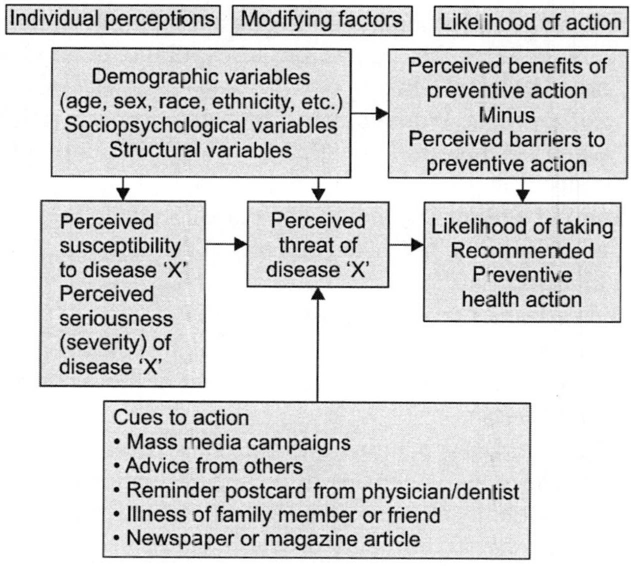

Fig. 23.2: Health belief model (Becker, 1974, 1988; Janz and Becker, 1984)

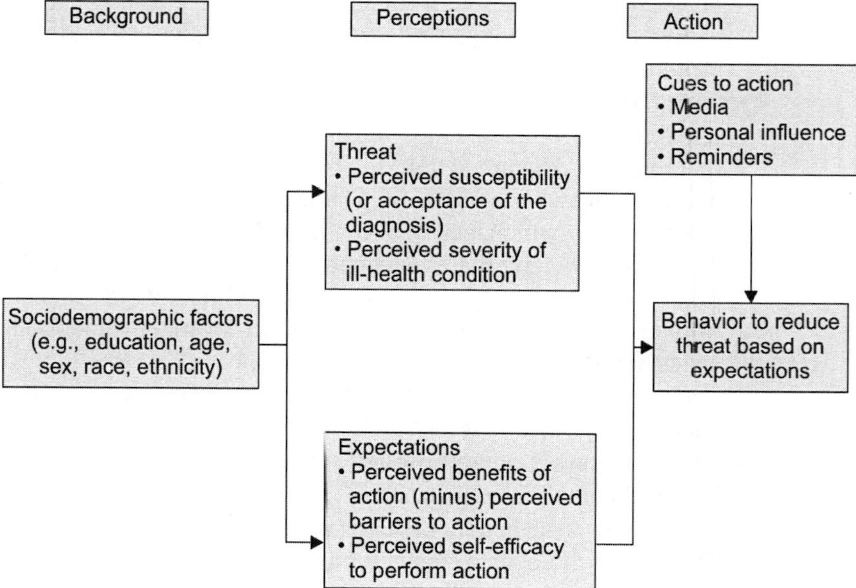

Fig. 23.3: Health belief model revised (Rosenstock, Strecher, and Becker, 1988)

APPLICATIONS

Nursing Research

- Components of HBM have been used for data collection in various researches.
- Hak-Seon Kim, Joo Ahn, and Jae-Kyung No (2012) were applied HBM in college students to investigate how university students' nutrition beliefs influence their health behavioral intention.

Nursing Education

- By providing discharge education to the patient regarding the importance of follow-up monitoring; this intervention may have positive effect on the quality of life and it help to prevent a readmission to the hospital. The patient needs to be accepting of the belief that post discharge nursing services in conjunction with self-efficacy may provide him or her with an improved quality of life.
- Education should be provided to ensure the patient understands the seriousness of disease states and its relation to his or her comorbidities.
- Morton (2008) used the HBM in the expansion and application of a health education program for school children.
- Ghaffari, Esmaillzadeh, Tavassoli, and Hassanzadeh (2012), uses HBM to give health education program in changing the behaviors of female adolescents to reduce the risk for osteoporosis was more effective.

Nursing Practice

- Health Belief Model has been used for nursing practice in different settings. It can be used in community as well as in clinical setting.
- Gutierrez and Long (2011), evaluated the accuracy of HBM scales that were designed to figure out what each of the HBM domains were for people with diabetes and serious mental illnesses (SMI).
- Kara, B, and Acikel, C (2009) analyze health beliefs on practicing breast self examination (BSE) among Turkish mothers and their daughters, who were nursing students.
- According to De Chesnay and Anderson (2012), the HBM has been useful for the identification of individuals who engage in behaviors relevant to primary and secondary prevention.

LIMITATIONS OF HEALTH BELIEF MODEL

Limitations of the Model Include the Following

- It does not consider a person's attitudes, beliefs, or other individual determinants that dictate a person's acceptance of a health behavior.
- It does not take into account behaviors that are habitual and thus may inform the decision-making process to accept a recommended action (e.g. smoking).

- It does not take into account behaviors that are performed for non-health related reasons such as social acceptability.
- It does not include environmental or economic factors that may also affect the recommended action.
- It assumes that everyone has access to equal amounts of information on the illness or disease.
- It assumes that cues to action are widely prevalent in encouraging people to act and that 'health' actions are the main goal in the decision-making process.
- It does not have predictive power.
- It is difficult to be tested.
- It is not suit for long-term behavioral change.

Critique of the HBM

- Health Belief Model only emphasis on the individual not give importance to social and economic factors.
- The absence of a role for emotional factors, such as fear and denial.
- Alternative factors may predict health behavior, such as outcome expectancy (whether the person feels they will be healthier as a result of their behavior) and self-efficacy.

PRACTICAL APPLICATION OF HEALTH BELIEF MODEL

Mr Rajesh, 28 years who is an engineer organizes immunization for his child who is 2 days old. Apply HBM (Fig. 23.4).

Health Belief Model—Revised (Rosenstock, Strecher, and Becker, 1988)

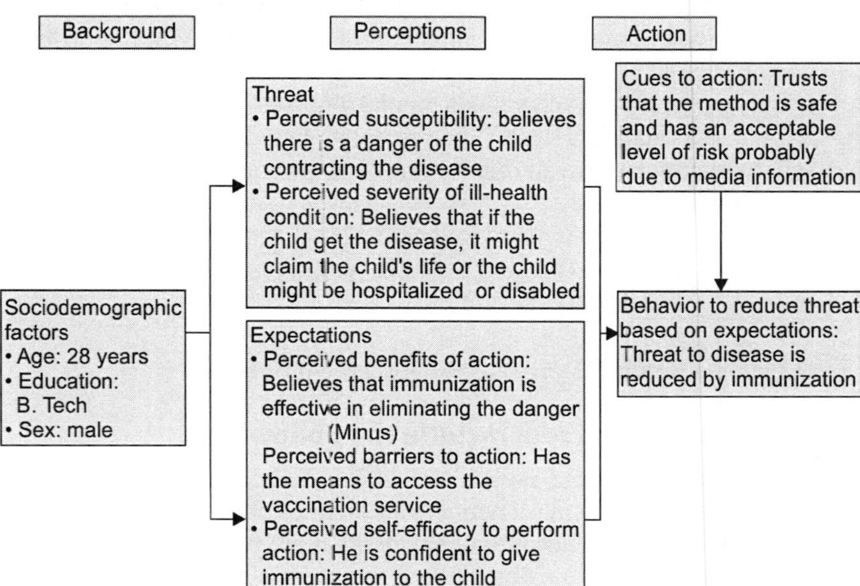

Fig. 23.4: Mr Rajesh as per health belief model

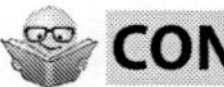 CONCLUSION

The HBM derives from psychological and behavioral theory with the foundation that the two components of health-related behavior are the desire to avoid disease; and, the belief that a specific health action will prevent, or cure, disease. Ultimately, an individual's course of action often depends on the person's perceptions of the benefits and barriers related to health behavior. The HBM is used to encourage healthy behavior among individuals in order to avoid negative health outcomes. A person must assess their perceptions of susceptibility and severity of developing a disease.

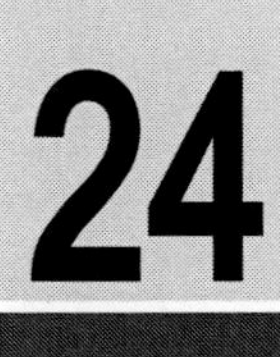

24 Nola J Pender: Health Promotion Model

'I believe that future will be very bright and productive for nurses who direct their careers toward understanding disease prevention and health promotion processes.'

–Nola J Pender

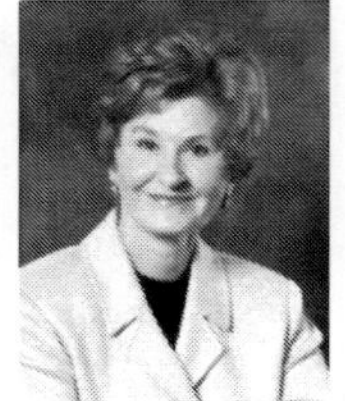

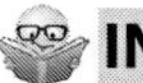 INTRODUCTION

The health promotion model (HPM) proposed by Nola J Pender (1982; revised in 1996) was designed to be a *complementary counterpart to models of health protection.* Health promotion means give awareness to people to choose healthy lifestyle and encouraging them to do things themselves. To achieve this, one should focus on health promoting strategies, such as daily physical activity, healthy nutrition, stress reduction or avoid the use of tobacco, alcohol or drugs.

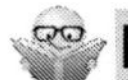 BIOGRAPHY

Pender was born in 1941 in Lansing, Michigan. Her parents were strong supporters of women education. She developed interest in nursing profession when she observed the nursing care given to her hospitalized aunt at the age of seven.

Educational Achievements

- Pender received her diploma from School of Nursing at West Suburban Hospital in Oak, Illinois in 1962.
- In 1964 Pender completed her BSN at Michigan State University in East Lansing.
- In 1965 she completed her MA in Human Growth and development from Michigan State University.
- She completed her PhD in Psychology and Education in 1969 at Northwestern University in Evanston, Illinois.
- Hon. Doctor of Science, Widener University, Chester, Pennsylvania in 1992.

Other Achievements

- Pender's Health promotion in Nursing Practice (4th edition) got ANA Book of the year Award for contribution to community health Nursing.

- She served as distinguished scholar at a number of universities.
- She received the alumni award from Michigan State University and holds an honorary degree from Widener University for her contribution to nursing research and health promotion.
- Midwest Nursing Research Society award for her contribution to research and research leadership.
- American Psychological Association award for contribution to nursing and health psychology.
- She was honored by the school of Nursing with the Mae Edna Doyle award for her excellence in teaching in 1998.
- She is a past president of the American Academy of Nursing and also served as president of the Midwest Nursing Research Society.
- She was a charter member of the National Advisory Council on Nursing Research.
- She is a member of the Board of Directors of research, America.
- In 1998, she was appointed to a 4 years term on the US Preventive Services Task Force.
- She serves on the Executive Committee of Building Health Promotion into the National Agenda.

Concepts of HPM

- *Person:* A biopsychosocial organism, i.e. partially shaped by the environment but also seeks to create an environment in which inherent and acquired human potential can be fully expressed. Thus, the relationship between person and environment is reciprocal. Individual characteristics as well as life experiences shape behaviors including health behaviors.
- *Environment:* The social, cultural and physical context in which the life course unfolds. The environment can be manipulated by the individual to create a positive context of cues and facilitators for health-enhancing behaviors.
- *Nursing:* It is collaboration with individuals, families, and communities to create the most favorable conditions for the expression of optimal health and high-level well-being.
- *Health:* In reference to the individual is defined as the actualization of inherent and acquired human potential through goal-directed behavior, competent self-care, and satisfying relationships with others, while adjustments are made as needed to maintain structural integrity and harmony with relevant environments. Health is an evolving life experience. There are definitions for family health and community health that have been proposed by other authors.
- *Illnesses:* Discrete events throughout the life span of either acute or chronic duration that can hinder or facilitate one's continuing quest for health.

Components of Model

- ***Individual characteristics and experiences:***
  - *Prior related behavior:* Frequency of the same or similar health behavior in the past which directly or indirectly effect on health promotion.
  - *Personal factors (biological, psychological, sociocultural)*: General characteristics of the individual that influence health behavior, such as age, gender, BMI, self-esteem, personality structure, race, ethnicity, education, and socioeconomic status.
- ***Behavior-specific cognitions and affect:***
  - *Perceived benefits of action:* Perceptions of the positive or reinforcing consequences of undertaking a health behavior. Prior positive experience with the behavior is a motivational factor.
  - *Perceived barriers to action:* Perceptions of the blocks, hurdles, and personal costs of undertaking a health behavior. It affect the health promoting behavior by decreasing individual commitment to a plan of action.
  - *Perceived self-efficacy:* Judgment of personal capability to organize and execute a particular health behavior; self-confidence in performing the health behavior successfully. Perceived high self-efficacy help to reduce the perceived barriers to action. People who have less confidence in their performance decrease their efforts for health promotion.
  - *Activity-related affect:* Subjective feeling states or emotions occurring prior to, during and following a specific health behavior. It affect perceived self efficacy that means more positive subjective feeling help to achieve more self efficacy.
  - *Interpersonal influences (primary sources are family, peers, providers):* Norms, social support, role models - perceptions concerning the behaviors, beliefs, or attitudes of relevant others in regard to engaging in a specific health behavior.
  - *Situational influences (options available, demand characteristics, esthetics features of the environment):* Perceptions of the compatibility of life context or the environment with engaging in a specific health behavior. It has direct or indirect effect on health behavior. If one has good options, safe and interesting environment helps in promoting health behavior.
  - *Commitment to a plan of action:* Intention to carry out a particular health behavior including the identification of specific strategies lead to implementation of health behavior.
  - *Immediate competing demands and preferences:* Alternative behaviors that intrude into consciousness as possible courses of action just prior to the intended occurrence of a planned health behavior.

- ***Behavioral outcome-health promoting behavior:***
  Health promoting behavior: The desired behavioral end point or outcome of health decision-making and preparation for action (*See* Flowchart on next page).

HEALTH PROMOTION MODEL ASSUMPTIONS

The HPM is based on the following assumptions, which reflect both nursing and behavioral science perspectives:

- One seeks to create conditions of living through which he/she can express his/her unique human health potential.
- People have the capacity for reflective self-awareness, including assessment of their own competencies.
- Person's value growth in directions viewed as positive and attempts to achieve a personally acceptable balance between change and stability.

Health Promotion Model

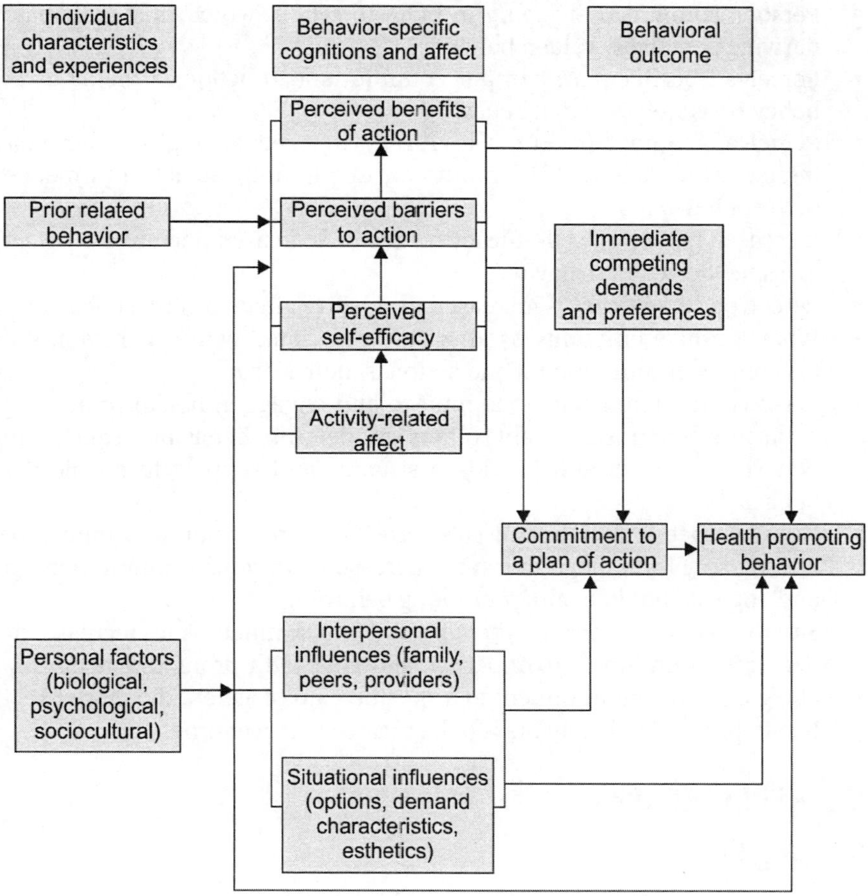

Fig. 24.1: Health promotion model

- One seeks to actively regulate his/her own behavior.
- Individuals in all their biopsychosocial complexity interact with the environment, progressively transforming the environment and being transformed over time.
- Health professionals constitute a part of the interpersonal environment, which exerts influence on persons throughout their lifespan.
- For behavior change, self-initiated reconfiguration of person-environment interactive patterns is essential.

HEALTH PROMOTION MODEL THEORETICAL PROPOSITIONS

Theoretical statements derived from the model provide a basis for investigative work on health behaviors. The HPM is based on the following theoretical propositions:

- Prior behavior and inherited and acquired characteristics influence beliefs, affect, and performance of health-promoting behavior.
- Persons commit to engaging in behaviors from which they anticipate deriving personally valued benefits.
- Perceived barriers can hamper commitment to action, a mediator of behavior as well as actual behavior.
- Perceived competence or self-efficacy to execute a given behavior increases the likelihood of commitment to action and actual performance of the behavior.
- Increased perceived self-efficacy results in decreased perceived barriers to a specific health behavior.
- Perceived self-efficacy is increased by positive affect toward a behavior.
- When positive emotions or affect are associated with a behavior, the probability of commitment and action is increased.
- Persons are more likely to commit to and engage in health-promoting behaviors when significant others model the behavior, expect the behavior to occur, and provide assistance and support to enable the behavior.
- Families, peers, and health care providers are important sources of interpersonal influence that may increase or decrease commitment to and engagement in health promoting behavior.
- Situational influences in the external environment can increase or decrease commitment to or participation in health-promoting behavior.
- The greater the commitment to a specific plan of action, the more likely health promoting behaviors is to be maintained over time.

APPLICATIONS

Nursing Practice

- Community health care setting is the best path in preventing disease and promoting health. Community program may be focused on activities to improve the wellness of the people by using Pender's HPM.

- In clinical setting also nurses can use Pender's HPM and give awareness to relatives of patients. Also she can educate clients to be effective health care consumers.
- Nurse can assist clients, families, and communities to develop and choose health promoting options.
- To use the latest knowledge about behavior change and determinants of particular health or risky behaviors to develop anticipatory guidance and counseling protocols.

Nursing Education

- Nurses can apply promotion model in giving health education to patients.
- Also nurses can use this model to prevent further complication of the disease. Thus can prevent worsening of that disease.
- This model could be a basis for structuring nursing protocols and interventions.
- The American Association of Colleges of Nursing which accredits Baccalaureate and Masters Nursing programs includes health promotion, risk reduction and disease prevention as core knowledge.
- An accreditation organization, the ACCN (2008) for baccalaureate nursing programs which has a health promotion essential. This essential includes an education outcomes that requires nursing programs to prepare students to provide input regarding the development of policies to promote health, provide health teaching and health counseling, identify environmental factors that affect current or future health problems, and assess protective and predictive factors which influence the health of individuals, groups, and communities (AACN, 2008).

Nursing Research

- Pender's HPM has been used in many research works and has always been found testable and applicable in research.
- Research helps nurse to develop a systematic problem-solving approach to improve and develop strategies to promote good health to individual.
- The HPM synthesizes research findings from nursing, psychology and public health into an explanatory model of health behavior that still must undergo further testing.

Limitations

- There are some factors than can be modified, such as biological (*example:* Body mass index), psychological (*example:* Self-motivation) and sociocultural factors (*example:* Education) that are predictive in given behaviors.
- The theory is focused on individual setting.

Critique of the HPM

- Clarity of the theory high level of logical concepts.
- The theory is very complex multiple phenomena involved.
- The theory is very easily generalized.
- Can be used in any health care setting.
- Large circle of contagiousness, very generalizable.
- Accessibility with modern technology the theory is very easily accessed, and has been used internationally.
- Useful in practice useful in research, useful in education, useful in guiding, and describing nursing care.

PRACTICAL APPLICATION OF HEALTH PROMOTION MODEL

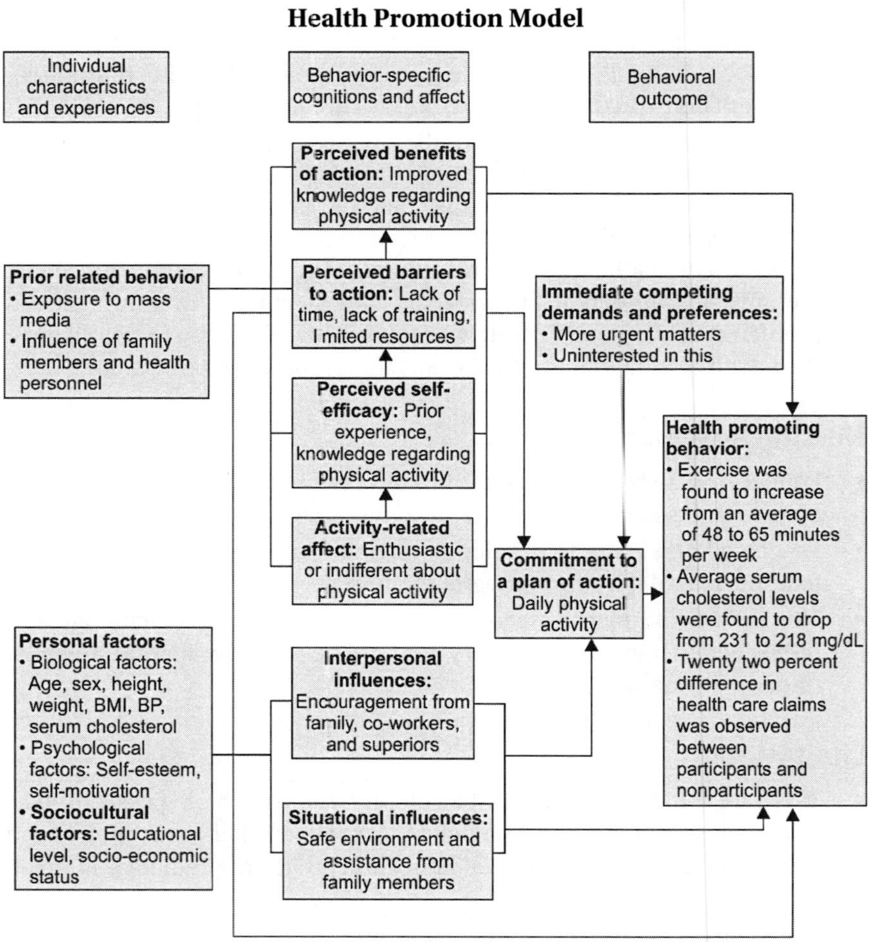

Fig. 24.2: Practical application of health promotion model

An occupational health nurse was interested in improving the health status of employees through implementation of a fitness program, such as worksite class (suggestions for incorporating physical activity into routine activities, such as walking and climbing stairs). A baseline assessment of employee was offered to them. The HPM-based assessment made by the nurse and given to the employee. And also she measured the physical measurements including height, weight, BMI, BP, and serum cholesterol level. Employee health care claims were also monitored. After 6 months period, the survey and physical measures were re-administered to employees, and result were compared. Moderate reductions in employee perceptions of barriers to exercise and situational influences on exercise were achieved. Employee participation in exercise was found to increase from an average of 48 to 65 minutes per week and average serum cholesterol levels were found to drop from 231 to 218 mg/dL. Twenty-two percent difference in health care claims was observed between participants and nonparticipants.

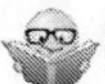 CONCLUSION

Prevention is better than cure. Thus, health promotion valued much. Health promotion model has given health care a new direction. According to Pender, Health promotion and disease prevention should be the primary focus in health care. Health promotion model focused on health promoting behaviors rather than health protection or illness prevention behaviors.

25 Hildegard E Peplau: Interpersonal Relations

'Nursing is an interpersonal process of therapeutic interactions between an individual who is sick or in need of health services and a nurse especially educated to recognize, respond to the need for help.'

–Hildegard E Peplau

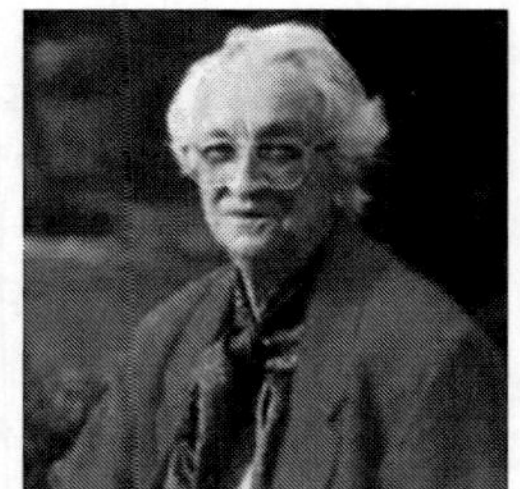

INTRODUCTION

Hildegard E Peplau is known as the mother of psychiatric nursing. The need for a partnership between nurse and client is essential for nursing practice. This helps nurses and health care providers to develop more therapeutic interventions in the clinical setting. Through these, Peplau developed her *'Interpersonal Relations Theory'* in 1952, mainly influenced by Henry Stack Sullivan, Percival Symonds, Abraham Maslow, and Neal Elgar Miller. Peplau's theory is also known as *psychodynamic nursing*, which is the understanding of one's own behavior.

Biography

- Hildegard E Peplau was born on September 1, 1909 in Reading, Pennsylvania.
- She was the second daughter of six children born to immigrant parents of German decent, Gustav and Ottylie Peplau.
- She died peacefully in her sleep 89 years later on March 17, 1999 in her home in Sherman Oaks, California.

Achievements

- In 1931, she graduated from Pottstown, Pennsylvania School of Nursing.
- In 1943, she completed her BA in interpersonal psychology from Bennington College, Vermont.
- She received MA in psychiatric nursing from Teachers College, Columbia, New York, in 1947 and EdD in curriculum development from Columbia in 1953.
- She received honorary Doctoral degrees during her prestigious career from the following universities: Alfred, Duke, Indiana, Ohio State, Rutgers and the University of Ulster in Ireland.

- Professor emeritus from Rutgers University.
- She started first post baccalaureate program in psychiatric nursing.
- She published Interpersonal Relations in Nursing in 1952.
- She worked as executive director and president of ANA.
- She also worked with WHO, NIMH and Nurse Corps.

ASSUMPTIONS

The assumptions of Peplau's Interpersonal Relations Theory are:

- The kind of person that the nurse becomes makes a substantial differences in what each patient will learn as he or she receives nursing care.
- Nurse and patient can interact with each other.
- Peplau emphasized that both the patient and nurse mature as the through the therapeutic interaction.
- Fundamental nursing tools are communication and interviewing skills.
- Peplau said that nurses must clearly understand themselves to promote their client's growth and to avoid limiting client's choices to those that nurses value.
- 'Fostering personality development toward maturity is function of nursing and nursing education. Nursing uses principles and methods that guide the process oward resolution of interpersonal problems.'

PARADIGM OF PEPLAU'S THEORY

It includes human being, health, environment, and nursing:

- **Human being**
  - Human being is an organism that lives unstable equilibrium.
  - Human being is a developing organism that tries to reduce anxiety caused by needs.
  - The client is an individual with a felt need.
- **Health**
  - Within her model Peplau did not include an exact description of health.
  - She viewed health as 'a word symbol that implied forward movement of personality and other ongoing human processes in the direction of creative, constructive, productive, personal, and community living.'
- **Environment**
  - Peplau does not include environment.
  - It is the 'existing force outside the organism and in the context of culture, from which mores, customs, and belief are acquired.'
  - General conditions that are likely to lead health always include the interpersonal process.
  - But she does encourage the nurse to believe the patient's culture and mores when the patient adjusts to hospital routine.

- **Nursing**
  - Peplau explain nursing as 'a significant, therapeutic, interpersonal process.'
  - Nurses function cooperatively with other human processes that make health possible for individuals in communities.
  - 'Nursing is an educative instrument, a maturing force that aims to promote forward movement of personality in the direction of creative, constructive, productive, personal, and community living.'

Concepts used by Peplau

- **Psychodynamic nursing**
  - Peplau consider psychodynamic nursing because her model evolves through this type of nursing.
  - 'Psychodynamic nursing is being able to understand one's own behavior to help others identify felt difficulties, and apply principles of human relations to the problems that arise at all level by experience.'
  - Peplau developed the model by defining the structural concepts of interpersonal process, which are the phases of the nurse patient relationship. This basic for psychodynamic nursing.
- **Nurse-patient relationship**
  - Peplau describes four phases of the nurse-patient relationship, i.e. orientation, identification, exploitation, and resolution.

Orientation	Problem defining phase
Identification	Selection of appropriate professional assistance
Exploitation	Use of professional assistance for problem solving alernatives
Resolution	Termnation of the professional relationships

Fig. 25.1: Phases of nurse patient realationship

  - Although these phases are separate, they overlap and occur over the time of the relationship.

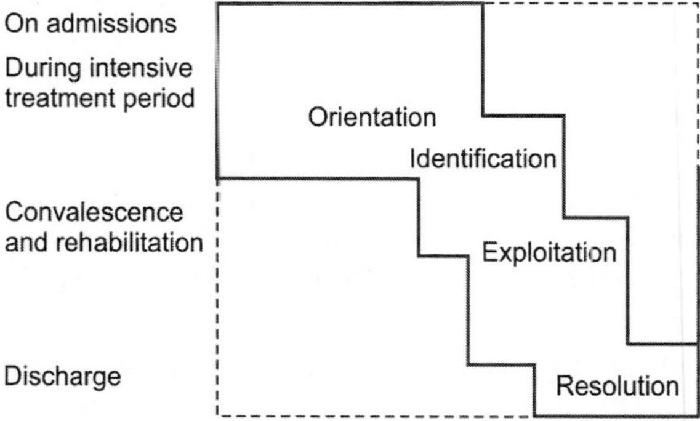

Fig. 25.2: Overlapping phases in nurse-patient relationship

- The factors influencing the blending nurse-patient relationship (NPR) is shown below.

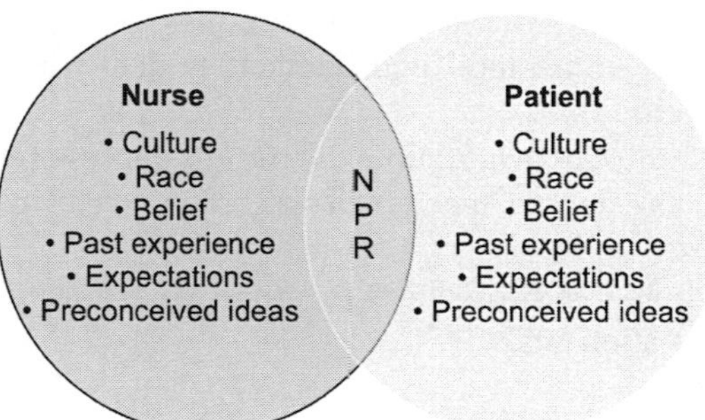

Fig. 25.3: Factors affecting nurse-patient ralationship

- Orientation
  - Problem defining phase.
  - Orientation phase starts when an individual felt need; seeks professional assistance and meets nurse as stranger.
  - The nurse helps the patient to recognize his problem and defining problem and deciding which type of service needed for him.
  - Client seeks assistance, conveys needs, and asks questions, shares preconceptions and expectations of past experiences to nurse.
  - Nurse responds, explains roles to client, helps to identify problems and to use available resources and services.
  - During this stage, it is important that a professional relationship should be established between nurse and client. This includes clarifying that the patient is the center of the relationship, and that all interactions are, and will be centered on helping the patient.
  - Trust begins to develop, and the client begins to recognize their role, the nurse's role, and the parameters and boundaries of their relationship.
- Identification
  - This phase begins when the patient works interdependently with the nurse, expresses feelings, and begins to feel stronger.
  - Selection of appropriate professional assistance.
  - Client begins to have a feeling of belonging and a capability to deal with the identified problem which decreases the feeling of helplessness and hopelessness.
- Exploitation:
  - Use of professional assistance for problem solving alternatives.
  - In the exploitation phase, the patient takes full use of the services offered and the client fully trusts the nurse.
  - The client takes advantages of services given are based on his needs and interests.

  - In this phase client feels as an integral part of the helping environment.
  - The principles of interview techniques must be used in order to explore, understand and adequately deal with the underlying problem.
  - Nurse must be aware about the various phases of communication, such as listening, teaching, and clarifying, etc. to give care to the patient.
  - The nurse and the client together work toward discharge and termination goals.
- Resolution:
  - Termination of the professional relationship.
  - In this phase, the patient no longer needs professional services and gives up dependent behavior. The relationship ends.
  - The client's needs have already been met by the collaborative effect of client and nurse.
  - In this phase, termination of their therapeutic relationship and dissolve the links between them.
  - Sometimes may be difficult for both nurse and client as psychological dependence persists.
  - Patient drifts away and breaks bond with nurse and healthier emotional balance is demonstrated and both nurse and client become mature individuals.

- **Nursing roles**
  - Peplau describes six nursing roles that emerge in the various phases of the nurse-patient relationship.

    a. **Stranger role**
    - Peplau describes that when the nurse meet the client first, they are thought to be strangers to one another. Therefore, the client should be treated with much respect, courtesy and equally as anybody else by the nurse.
    - The nurse should not anticipate the client or give assumptions on the patient but take him as he is.
    - The nurse should treat the client as emotionally stable, unless evidence states otherwise.

    b. **Resource role**
    - The nurse provides answers to questions manly the health related information.
    - The resource person is also give relaying information to the client regarding the treatment and plan of care.
    - Usually the questions are arisen from larger problems therefore, the nurse would determine what type of response is appropriate for constructive learning whether giving straightforward answers or providing information on counseling.

c. **Teaching role**
   - The teaching role is a role is the combination of all roles.
   - Teacher who imparts knowledge according to a need or interest.
   - Peplau considered that there are two types of teaching role which are: *Instructional and experimental.* The instructional consists of giving a wide variety of information, i.e., given to the clients and experimental is using the experience of the learner as a starting point to later form products of learning which the client makes about their experiences.

d. **Counseling role**
   - Peplau considered that counseling has the biggest role in psychiatric nursing.
   - The councilor role helps the client to understand and remember what is going on and what is happening to them in current life situations.
   - The nurse also provide guidance and encouragement to make changes in clients.

e. **Surrogate role**
   - The client is casts the nurse in the surrogate role.
   - The nurse's behaviors and attitudes create a feeling tone for the client that cause feelings that were generated in a previous relationship.
   - The nurse helps the client to recognize the similarities and differences between the nurse and the past relationship.
   - The nurse helps to clarify the client about domains of dependence interdependence and independence and acts behalf as an advocate.

f. **Leadership role**
   - As a leader, the nurse helps the client to assume maximum responsibility for meeting treatment goals in a mutually satisfying way. The nurse helps the client to meet these goals through cooperation and active participation with the nurse.
   - The nurse gives direction to the client or group.

- **Psychobiological experiences**
  - Peplau describes four psychological experiences: Need, Frustration, Conflict, and anxiety.
  - These experiences provide energy that transformed into some form of action.
  - Peplau uses non-nursing theoretical concepts to identify and explain these experiences that compel destructive or constructive responses from nurses and patients.
  - This understanding provides a basis for goal formation and nursing interventions.

Continum showing changing aspect of nurse-patient relationship

Patient: Personal goals —————————— Patient

Entirely separate goals and interests both are strangers to each other	Individual preconceptions on the meaning of the medical problem, the roles of each in the problematic situation	Partially mutual and individual understanding of the medical problem	Mutual understanding of the nature of the problem, roles of nurse and patient, and requirements of nurse and patient in the solution of the problem common, shared health goals	Collaborative efforts directed toward solving the problem together productively

Nurse: Professional goals —————————— Nurse

 INTERPERSONAL THEORY AND NURSING PROCESS

Peplau's phases and interpersonal process can be compared to the nursing process. Both Peplau's Interpersonal Relations Theory and the Nursing Process are sequential and focus on therapeutic relationship Both use observation communication and recording as basic tools for nursing practice.

Comparison between nursing process and Peplau's interpersonal phases

Nursing process	Peplau's interpersonal phases
Assessment • Data collection and analysis-continuous • May or may not be a felt need.	**Orientation** • Data collection-non continuous • Felt need • Need is defined
Nursing diagnosis and planning • Mutually set goals	**Identification** • Interdependent goal setting
Implementation • Plans initiated and move toward the achievement of mutually set goals • May be accomplished by patient, (health care professional) nurse, or significant other (relatives).	**Exploitation** • Patient actively seeking and drawing for help • Patient initiated

Contd...

Contd...

Nursing process	Peplau's interpersonal phases
Evaluation • Based on mutually established expected behaviors • May led to termination of relationship and initiation of new plans	**Resolution** • Occurs after other phases are completed successfully • Leads to termination of relationship

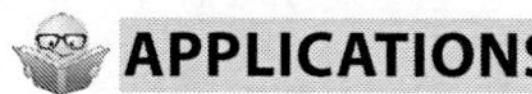

APPLICATIONS

Nursing Education

- Peplau's theoretical ideas, particularly her definition of nursing and nursing process, psychodynamic methods, have become a part of the collective culture of the discipline of nursing.
- She designed and published her model in 1952, 1957, and 1962 with a particular emphasis on psychiatric nursing.

Nursing Research

- Many researchers use Peplau's theory to guide program of study that applies this theory to clinical practice.
- Penckofer S, Byrn M, Mumby P, Ferrans CE (2011) uses Peplau's theory of interpersonal relations for improving subject recruitment, retention, and participation in research.

Nursing Practice

- Peplau brought 'a new perspective, a new approach, and a theoretically based foundation for nursing practice for therapeutic work with patients'.
- Her work is responsible for a second order change in the nursing culture.
- Clinicians continue to use Peplau's model extensively.
- Ann R Peden, RN; DSN uses Peplau's theory to describe the process of recovering in women who have been depressed.

Limitations

- Health promotion and maintenance were less given importance in the theory.
- The theory cannot be used in a client who does not have a felt need, such as with withdrawn patients and unconscious patient.
- Personal space considerations, community and social service resources are considered less in this theory.
- Some areas in this theory are not specific enough to generate hypothesis.

Critiquing the Theory

- *Clarity:* Clear; easily understandable. She clearly defines the theory's basic assumptions and key concepts.

- *Simplicity:* Simple; the theory has few concepts and relationships.
- *Empirical precision:* Orlando's theory is used in many research work has been found testable and applicable in research. This theory provides a theory based on reality. The relationship between the theory and empirical data allows other scientists to validate and verify the theory.
- *Generality:* Focuses on a limited number of situations; it could be modified and can be used in other nursing situations and other professional fields. But this theory only applied where nurse-patient relationship is possible. Its use is limited with the comatose, newborn patients.

PRACTICAL APPLICATION OF PEPLAU'S INTERPERSONAL THEORY

Mr Suresh, 28-year-old male who come to psychiatric clinic with his wife, has symptoms of anxiety and fatigue and with a history of substance abuse and alcohol abuse.

Assessment (orientation phase)	Nursing diagnosis	Planning (identification phase)	Implementation (exploitation phase)	Evaluation (resolution phase)
• The nurse works as a counselor to establish a relationship with Mr Suresh and his wife. • identify the problem	• Ineffective coping related to situational stressors	• Goal setting done along with the patient • Make the patient to do the breathing exercise • Do diversional therapy to divert his mind • Practice coping strategies	• Carried out plans mutually agreed upon • Made the patient to do breathing exercise • Provided non-pharmacological measures like diversion, massaging, reading articles • Taught coping strategies	• He expressed satisfaction when anxiety decreased

CONCLUSION

Peplau has developed a nursing model which is useful in variety of nursing field in which the nurse is engaged in a therapeutic relationship with the client. Peplau makes theoretical relationships throughout her book. In summarizing these relationships Peplau addresses the patient-nurse relationship. She present nursing as an educative force that uses the experiential learning method for both patient and nurse.

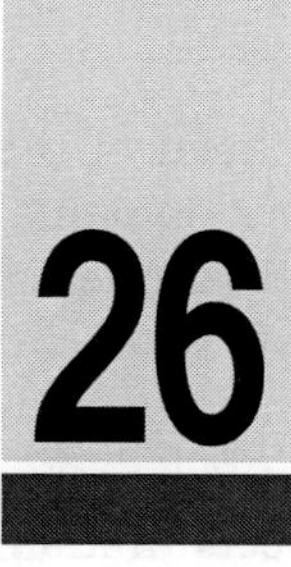

26 Larry D Purnell: Purnell's Model for Cultural Competence

 INTRODUCTION

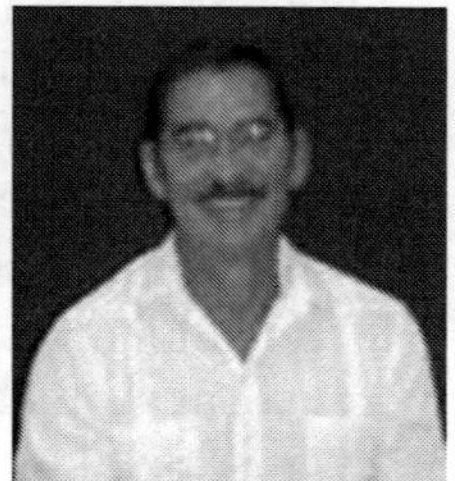

Larry D Purnell

The model consists of 12 domains with the primary and secondary characteristics of culture, which determine variations in values, beliefs, and practices of an individual's cultural heritage. All health care providers in any practice setting can use the model, which makes it especially desirable in today's team-oriented health care environment.

Purposes of the Purnell Model

- Provide a framework for all health care providers to learn concepts and characteristics of culture.
- Define circumstances that affect a person's cultural worldview in the context of historical perspectives.
- Provide a model that links the most central relationships of culture.
- Interrelate characteristics of culture to promote congruence and to facilitate the delivery of consciously sensitive and competent health care.
- Provide a framework that reflects human characteristics, such as motivation, intentionality, and meaning.
- Provide a structure for analyzing cultural data.
- View the individual, family, or group within their unique ethnocultural environment.

Major concepts: There are 12 cultural domains.

1. **Overview/heritage:** Concepts related to country of origin, current residence, and the effects of the topography of the country of origin and current residence, economics, politics, reasons for emigration, educational status, and occupations.
2. **Communication:** Concepts related to the dominant language and dialects; contextual use of the language; paralanguage variations, such as voice volume, tone, and intonations; and the willingness to share thoughts and feelings. Nonverbal communications, such as the use of eye contact, facial expressions, touch, body language, spatial distancing practices, and acceptable greetings; temporality in terms of past, present, or future worldview orientation; clock *vs* social time; and the use of names are important concepts.

3. **Family roles and organization:** Concepts related to the head of the household and gender roles; family roles, priorities, and developmental tasks of children and adolescents; child-rearing practices; and roles of the ages and extended family members. Social status and views toward alternative lifestyles, such as single parenting, sexual orientation, childless marriages, and divorce are also included in the domain.
4. **Workforce issues:** Concepts related to autonomy, acculturation, assimilation, gender roles, ethnic communication styles, individualism, and health care practices from the country of origin.
5. **Bicultural ecology:** Includes variations in ethnic and racial origins, such as skin coloration and physical differences in body stature; genetic, heredity, endemic, and topographical diseases; and differences in how the body metabolizes drugs.
6. **High-risk behaviors:** Includes the use of tobacco, alcohol and recreational drugs; lack of physical activity; nonuse of safety measures such, as seatbelts and helmets; and high-risk sexual practices.
7. **Nutrition:** Includes having adequate food; the meaning of food; food choices, rituals, and taboos; and how food and food substances are used during illness and for health promotion and wellness.
8. **Pregnancy and childbearing:** Includes fertility practices; methods for birth control; views toward pregnancy; and prescriptive, restrictive, and taboo practices related to pregnancy, birthing, and postpartum treatment.
9. **Death rituals:** Includes how the individual and the culture view death, rituals and behaviors to prepare for death, and burial practices. Bereavement behaviors are also included in this domain.
10. **Spirituality:** Includes religious practices and the use of prayer, behaviors that give meaning to life, and individual sources of strength.
11. **Health care practices:** Includes the focus of health care, such as acute or preventive; traditional, magico-religious, and biomedical beliefs; individual responsibility for health; self-medication practices; and views toward mental illness, chronicity, and organ donation and transplantation. Barriers to health care and one's response to pain and the sick role are included in this domain.
12. **Health care practitioner:** Concepts include the status, use, and perceptions of traditional, magico-religious, and allopathic biomedical health care providers. In addition, the gender of the health care provider may have significance.

Concepts of Cultural Consciousness

- ***Variant cultural characteristics:*** Age, generation, nationality, race, color, gender, religion, educational status, socioeconomic status, occupation, military status, political beliefs, urban *vs* rural residence, enclave identity, marital status, parental status, physical characteristics, sexual orientation, gender issues, and reason for migration.
- ***Unconsciously incompetent:*** Not being aware that one is lacking knowledge about another culture.

- ***Consciously incompetent:*** Being aware that one is lacking knowledge about another culture.
- ***Consciously competent:*** Learning about the client's culture, verifying generalizations about the client's culture, and providing culturally specific interventions.
- ***Unconsciously competent:*** Automatically providing culturally congruent care to clients of diverse cultures.

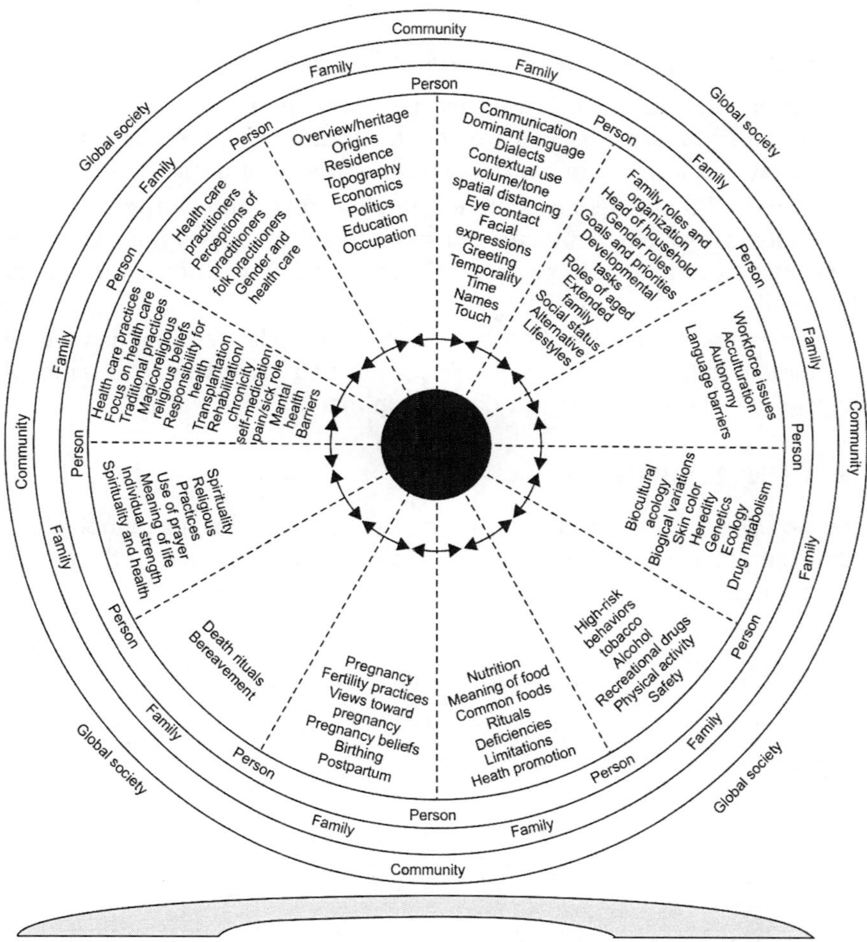

Fig. 26.1: Purnell's model for cultural competence

The model is a circle, with an outlying rim representing global society, a second rim representing community, a third rim representing family, and an inner rim representing the person. The interior of the circle is divided into12 pie-shaped wedges depicting cultural domains and their concepts. The dark center of the circle represents unknown phenomena. Along the bottom of the model is a jagged line representing the nonlinear concept of cultural consciousness.

Metaparadigm Concepts

Person: A biopsychosociocultural being who is constantly adapting to his or her environment.

Health: A state of wellness as defined by people within their ethnocultural group. Health generally includes physical, mental, and spiritual states.

Community: A group of people having a common interest or identity and living in a specified locality.

Application of Purnell's Model for Cultural Competence

Education: This model has used by the nurses, nutritionists, physicians, physical therapists, and social workers for staff development and various courses. It also acts as a framework to study various cultural studies.

Practice: This model has its applicability in all the health care professionals due to its various environmental contexts. This can act as a framework for deciding assessment tools, planning and implementing various strategies to the population.

Research: A majority of health care professionals are using this model in their researchers. The primary and secondary characteristics of this model are used to collect demographic data of population.

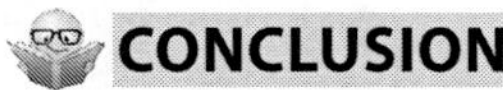

CONCLUSION

The model of cultural competence is proposed as an organizing framework to guide cultural competence among multidisciplinary members of the health care team in a variety of primary secondary, and tertiary settings.

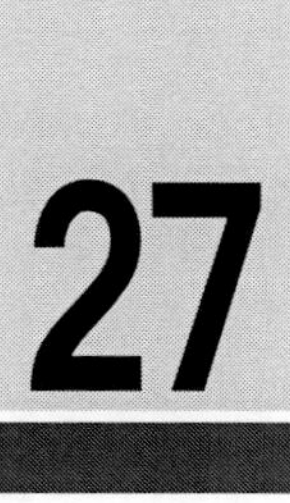

Barbara Resnick: Middle Range Nursing Theory of Self-Efficacy

INTRODUCTION

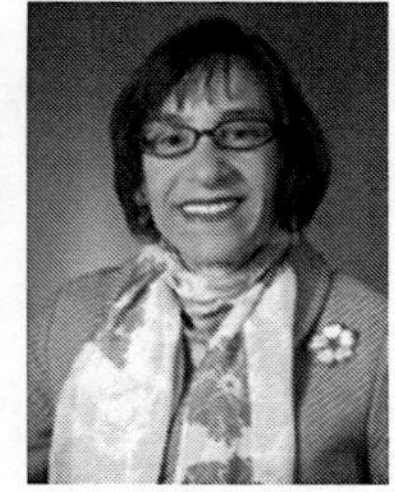

Barbara Resnick

This theory attempts to predict and explain behavior using several key concepts, such as self-efficacy expectations, outcome expectations, and incentives. This states that self-efficacy expectations and outcome expectations are not only influenced by behavior, but also by verbal encouragement, physiological sensations and exposure to role models or self-modeling.

Biography

- She graduated in Nursing from University of Connecticut.
- She received Masters degree in Nursing in Gerontological Nurse Clinician/Nurse Practitioner program from University of Pennsylvania.
- University of Maryland conferred her PhD in Nursing.
- She worked in different caders in the University of Maryland.
- She published numerous research articles and wrote a book titled *Restorative Care Nursing*.
- She is a recipient of various awards in research and clinical excellence.
- Her research interest is the motivation of elderly people in engaging in activities.

Assumptions

- We have powerful cognitive or symbolizing capabilities that allow for the creation of internal models of experience, the development of innovative courses of action, the hypothetical testing, and the communication.
- Environmental events, inner personal factors (cognition, emotion, and biological events), and behaviors are reciprocal influences.
- Self and personality are socially embedded.
- We are capable of self-regulation.

Major Concepts

Self-efficacy: It is an individual view about his or her to organize and execute course of action.

Outcome expectations are the judgments of an individual toward outcome of the successful completion of tasks. Those individuals who have high expected outcome are supposed to show higher adherence toward the treatment plan. Exposure to enactive mastery experiences, such as participation in an exercise class, is the most common intervention used to strengthen efficacy expectations in older adults.

Self-efficacy expectations: Which are the individuals' beliefs in their capabilities to perform a course of action to attain a desired outcome.

Sources of self-efficacy judgment: Barbara identified an individual judgment about his or her self-efficacy is based on four main informational sources (Fig. 27.1).

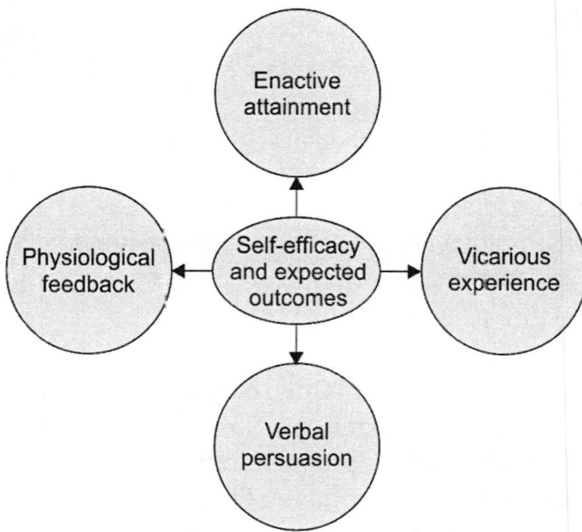

Fig. 27.1: Sources of self-efficacy judgment

- **Enactive attainment:** This is the most influential source in which an individual actually perform an activity. This performance strengthens his or her self-efficacy and expectations. However, ability, difficulty of the task, efforts and situation variables can influence this source.
- **Vicarious experience:** This is an experience in which an individual visualize the other people when performing the similar task. It can be influenced by the interest of an individual.
- **Verbal persuasion:** It is persuading an individual that he or she can perform and get mastery over the particular activities. It is found very effective in avoiding the healthy risky behavior among chronically ill patients. Verbal persuasion is a less potent source of enduring change in self-efficacy expectancy than performance experiences and vicarious experiences.
- **Physiological feedback:** Individuals believe on physiological indicators in order to assess their abilities. Physiological indicants of self-efficacy expectancy, however, extend beyond autonomic arousal. For example, in activities involving strength and stamina, such as exercise and athletic performances, perceived efficacy is influenced by such experiences as fatigue and pain.

Application of Theory of Self-Efficacy

Nursing education: This theory has been a framework for many training program for the elderly people in implementing physical activities. It is also used to teach and assist nurses for giving restorative nursing care.

Nursing practice: All the sources of self-efficacy judgment make the nurses to understand the patients correctly. These methods can effectively apply in clinical areas to strengthen the self-efficacy of patients.

Nursing research: This theory has been used in various researches mainly to improve the clinical practice and training of nurses.

CONCLUSION

Self-efficacy theory asserts that efficacy expectations determine approach behavior and physiological arousal of phobics as well as numerous other clinically important behaviors.

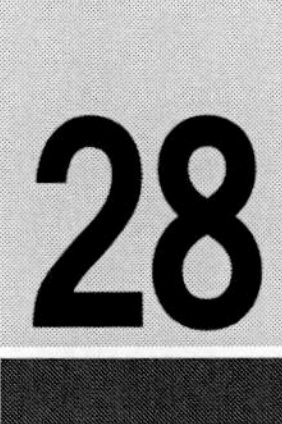

28 Ramona Thieme Mercer: Theory of Maternal Role Attainment

'The process of becoming a mother requires extensive psychological, social, and physical work. A woman experiences heightened vulnerability and faces tremendous challenges as she makes this transition. Nurses have an extraordinary opportunity to help women learn, gain confidence, and experience growth as they assume the mother identity'.

–Ramona Thieme Mercer

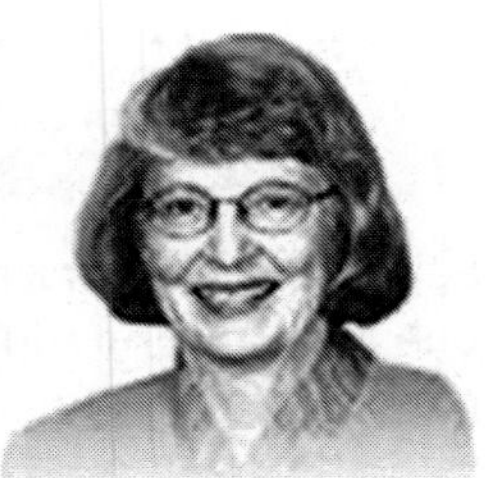

 **INTRODUCTION**

Ramona T Mercer developed Maternal Role Attainment Theory in the late nineteen sixties in order to achieve a strong, maternal identity in a woman's lifetime. She introduced the idea of Maternal Role Attainment while she was a Doctoral Scholar at the University of Pittsburgh and was inspired by her instructor and mentor, Reva Rubin. Since its beginning, she has revised and extended her theory process to 12 months postpartum and in 2004, changed the name as 'Maternal Role Attainment: Becoming a Mother'. Her concepts form a framework that centers on developing a strong bond between the mother and child and which enhance the role of motherhood.

Biography and Achievement

- She was born on October 4, 1929.
- She graduated in 1950 with her nursing diploma at the age of 21 from Saint Margaret's School of Nursing in Montgomery, Alabama.
- For the next 10 years she worked as a nurse, head nurse and instructor in pediatric and obstetrical nursing and in the field of contagious diseases.
- Her early nursing experience molded her interests toward pediatric and obstetrics.
- In 1960 she returned to school and earned an Undergraduate degree in nursing with distinction from the University of New Mexico, Albuquerque in 1962 and in 1964 earned her master's degree specializing in maternal-child nursing from Emory University.
- She continued pursuing her passion for maternity nursing and received her PhD from University of Pittsburgh in 1973.
- Then she moved to California and worked as a Nursing Professor at the University of California until she retired in 1987.

- She believes that 'theory building is a continual process' and so even after her retirement, she still continues to revise and clarify her work.
- She 1970's mainly focused on the needs of breastfeeding mothers, teenage mothers, postpartum illness, and mothers bearing children with defects.
- She also had a deep interest in the development of the maternal role as well as self-esteem and self-concept of mothers.
- During the span of Mercer's career, her work expanded further in the area of maternal-child nursing and she authored books, such as *Perspectives on Adolescent Health Care, Transitions in a Woman's Life,* and *Parents at Risk.*
- She has written of six books, published six book chapters and numerous journal articles.
- Throughout her career she has received numerous awards and is a member of several professional organizations and national committees.

CONCEPTS USED BY MERCER

The primary concept in Mercer's theory of Maternal Role Attainment (revised to 'Becoming a Mother' in her 1995 book 'Becoming a Mother: Research on Maternal Identity from Rubin to the Present') is that motherhood is a developmental and interactional process through which the mother and her child bond over time. She describes four distinct phases in the process, the names of which she revised in 2004.

- *Maternal role attainment:*
  - It is defined as an interactional and developmental process occurring over a period of time, in which the mother becomes attached to her baby, acquires competence in the care-taking tasks involved in the role, and expresses pleasure and satisfaction in the role.
  - 'The movement to the personal state in which the mother experiences a sense of harmony, confidence, and competence in how she performs the role is the end point of maternal role attainment.'
- *Maternal age:* Means chronological and developmental.
- *Perception of birth experience:* This means a woman's perception of her performance during intrapartum and birth.
- *Maternal identity:* It is defined as having an internalized view of the self as a mother.
- *Early maternal-infant separation:* Separation of infant from the mother after birth due to illness, prematurity, etc.
- *Self-esteem:* It is defined as an 'individual's perception of how others view ones and self-acceptance of the perception.'
- *Self-concept (self-regard):* According to Mercer self concept or self regard defined as 'The overall perception of self that includes self-satisfaction, self-acceptance, self-esteem, and congruence of discrepancy between self and ideal self.'

- *Flexibility:* According to her, one's role is not rigidly fixed. Therefore, who fills the roles is not important. 'Flexibility of childrearing attitudes increases with increased development...older mothers have the potential to respond less rigidly to their infants and to view each situation in respect to the unique nuances.'
- *Childrearing attitudes:* This means maternal attitudes or beliefs about childrearing.
- *Health status:* Mercer defined health status as 'The mother's and father's perception of their prior health, current health, health outlook, resistance-susceptibility to illness, health worry concern, sickness orientation and rejection of the sick role.'
- *Anxiety:* Anxiety is an attribute in which there is specific proneness to perceive stressful situations as dangerous or threatening, and as situation-specific state.
- *Depression:* Depression means 'Having a group of depressive symptoms, and in particular, the affective component of the depressed mood.'
- *Role strain (role coflict):* This means the conflict and difficulty felt by the mother in fulfilling the maternal role responsibility.
- *Gratification (satisfaction):* According to Mercer, gratification means the satisfaction, enjoyment, reward, or pleasure that a mother experiences in interacting with her infant, and in fulfilling the usual tasks inherent in mothering.
- *Attachment:* It is a component of the parental role and identity. Attachment is viewed as a process in which an enduring affectional and emotional commitment to a person is formed.
- *Infant temperament:* An easy *vs* a difficult temperament, it is related to whether the infant sends hard-to-read cues, leading to the feelings of incompetence and frustration in the mother.
- *Infant health status:* Mercer describes it is an illness which causes maternal-infant separation, interfering with the attachment process.
- *Infant characteristics:* Include temperament, appearance, and health status.
- *Infant cues:* Infant cues mean infant behaviors that elicit a response from the mother.
- *Family:* 'A dynamic system which includes subsystems—individuals (mother, father, fetus/infant) and dyads (mother-father, mother-fetus/infant, and father-fetus/infant) within the overall family system.'
- *Family functioning:* The one's view of the activities and relationships between the family and its subsystems and broader social units.
- *Father or intimate partner:* The father or intimate partner contributes to the process of maternal role attainment in a way that cannot be duplicated by any other individual. The father's interactions help diffuse tension and also helps in maternal role attainment.
- *Stress:* It is made up of positively and negatively perceived life events and environmental variables.

- *Social support:* This means 'the amount of help actually received, satisfaction with that help, and the persons (network) providing that help.'

  Four areas of social support are the following:

  a. *Emotional support:* Feeling loved, cared for, trusted, and understood.
  b. *Informational support:* This helps the individual help herself by providing information, i.e. useful in dealing with the problem and/or situation.
  c. *Physical support:* It is a direct kind of help.
  d. *Appraisal support:* A support that tells the role taker how she is performing in the role; it enables the person to evaluate herself in relationship to other's performance in the role.
- *Mother-father relationship:* This relationship means perception of the mate relationship that includes intended and actual values, goals, and agreements between the two. The maternal attachment to the infant develops within the emotional held of the parent's relationship.
- *Culture:* The total way of life learned and passed on from one generation to another generation.

MAJOR ASSUMPTIONS

According to Mercer these are the following assumptions which help in the maternal role attainment:

- A relatively stable core self, acquired through life long socialization, determines how a mother defines and perceives events; her perceptions of her infant's and others' responses to her mothering, with her life situation, are the real world to which she responds.
- The mother's developmental level and innate personality characteristics also influence her behavioral responses in addition to her socialization.
- The mother's role partner, her infant, will reflect the mother's competence in the mothering role through growth and development.
- The infant is considered an active partner in the maternal role-taking process, affecting and being affected by the role enactment.
- The father or mother's intimate partner contributes to role attainment in a way that cannot be duplicated by any other supportive persons.
- Maternal identity develops with maternal attachment and each depends on one other.

METAPARDIGM OF THE THEORY

Nursing

- Mercer does not define nursing but refers to nursing is a science, i.e. emerging from a 'turbulent adolescence to adulthood.'

- 'Nurses are the health professionals having the most sustained and intense interaction with mother in the maternity cycle.'
- Obstetric Nursing is the diagnosis and treatment of women's and men's responses to actual or potential health problems during antepartum, intrapartum, and the postpartum period.
- Mercer also emphasizes that the kind of help of a mother receives during antepartum, intrapartum and over the first year following delivery can have a lifelong term effects for her and child.

Person

- Mercer does not specifically define person or individual but refers to the 'self' or 'core-self'. According to her, self as separate from the roles that are played. The women interacts with her infant and with the father or her significant other; influential and is influenced by both of them.
- Through maternal individuation, a woman may regain her own 'personhood' as she extrapolates her 'self' from the mother-infant dyad.
- The core self evolves from a culture context and determines how situations are defined and shaped.

Health

- Mercer given most importance of health care during the child bearing and child-rearing process.
- The health status is an important indirect influence on satisfaction with relationships in antenatal families.
- She also defines health status as the parent's perception of their prior health, current health, health outlook, resistance, susceptibility to illness, health worry or concerns, sickness orientation and rejection to sick role.
- Health status of the newborn baby is the extent of disease present and infant health status by parental rating of overall health.

Environment

- Mercer's definition on environment is taken from Urie Bronfenbrenner's definition of the ecological environment.
- Development of role/individual cannot be considered apart from the environment. There is a mutual accommodation between the settings and relationships between settings are embedded.
- Mercer's model shows nesting of the mother and infant with the microsystem, mesosystem, and macrosystem. The model indicates the environmental factors such a social support, stress, and family functioning within the microsystem and environmental factors, such as work setting, school, and daycare impact role attainment. Stresses within the environment therefore, influence both maternal and parental role attainment and the developing their child.

 THEORETICAL ASSERTIONS (PROPOSED MODEL OF MATERNAL ROLE ATTAINMENT)

Mercer's model of maternal role attainment is placed within Urie Bronfenbrenner's nested cycle of the microsystem, mesosystem, and macrosystem:

- The microsystem is the immediate environment where maternal role attainment occurs. This indicates the family and factors, such as family functioning, mother-father relationships, social support, economic status, family valuess, and stress. The infant is an individual embedded within the family system. Most influential on maternal role attainment is the microsystem and attainment is achieved within this system through the interactions of father, mother and infant.
- The mesosystem encompasses, influences and delimits the microsystem and also interact with the individual in the microsystem and also. The mother-infant unit is not contained within the mesosystem, but the mesosystem may determine in part what happens to the developing maternal role and her child. It includes extended family, school, day care, work setting, church and other places of worship and other entities within the mother's more immediate community. The exosystem (the previously used term) is an extension of the mesosystem. It is the interrelationships of two or more settings or subsystems that more directly influences the women, such as interactions between works setting, daycare, local laws and rules, community, and church.
- The macrosystem means the general prototypes existing in a particular culture or transmitted cultural consistencies and which include the social, political and cultural influences on other two systems. In this macrosystem where the health care environment and the impact of current health care system on maternal role attainment originate.
- Maternal role attainment is a process and that follows four stages of role acquisition; these stages have been adapted from Thornton and Nardi's (1975) research. These four stages are indicated as microsystem within the evolving model of Maternal Role Attainment. The original model's four stage process are follows:
    a. *Anticipatory stage:* This stage begins during the antenatal period and which includes the initial social and psychological adjustments to pregnancy. The woman learns the expectations of the role, fantasizes about the role, related to the fetus in the uterus, and begins role play.
    b. *Formal stage:* This stage begins with the birth of the infant (intranatal) and includes learning and taking of the role of the mother. The Role behaviors are guided by formal, consensual expectations and others in the mother's social system.
    c. *Informal stage:* This stage begins as the mother develops unique way of dealing with the role ant that not influenced by her social system. The mother makes her new role fit within her existing lifestyle based on past experiences and future goals.

d. *Personal stage:* This stage begins as the woman internalizes her role. At this stage, the mother experiences harmony, confidence and competence in the way she performs the role and the maternal role is achieved.

- These four stages of role acquisition overlap and are altered as the infant grows as and develop. The final stage of maternal role identity may be attained in many period of time. The stages are influenced by social support, stress, family functioning, and the relationship between the parents or significant others.
- Mercer proposed that the term becoming mother more accurately reflected the process in her theory. This is because she believed that the previous term suggested an end point, whereas she believes the process is ongoing expansion of the self as a mother. Proposed changes in the names of the stages are the following (revised model-2004).
  - *Commitment, attachment, and preparation stage (pregnancy):* During pregnancy when the women makes psychological adjusts and prepares for the expectations of her new role.
  - *Acquaintance, practice, and physical restoration (first 2 weeks):* This begins with the infant's birth when the role of mother is assumed and learned in the contexts of her social system.
  - *Approaching normalization (second week to 4 months):* In the first few months of the infant's life where the mother makes her new role fit her lifestyle in a personal way instead of in context with a social system.
  - *Integration of maternal identity (Approximately 4 months):* When the mother internalizes her role and experiences a sense of harmony, competence and confidence which usually occurs about 4 months after birth.
- Both the mother's and the infant's traits and behaviors may influence maternal role identity and child outcome.
- Maternal traits and behaviors included in the model are empathy, sensitivity to child cues, self-esteem and self-concept, parenting received as a child, maturity and flexibility, attitude, pregnancy and birth experience, health, depression and role conflict/strain.
- Child traits having an impact on maternal role identity include temperament, ability to send cues, appearance, general characteristics, responsiveness, and stress.
- According to Mercer, the maternal role is achieved when the mother feels internal harmony with the role and its expectations and described three major components of the role:
  - Attachment to the child.
  - Gaining competence/confidence in mothering behaviors.
  - Expressing gratification in maternal-infant interactions.
- Outcome of the child includes cognitive/mental development behavior/attachment, health, and other social competence.

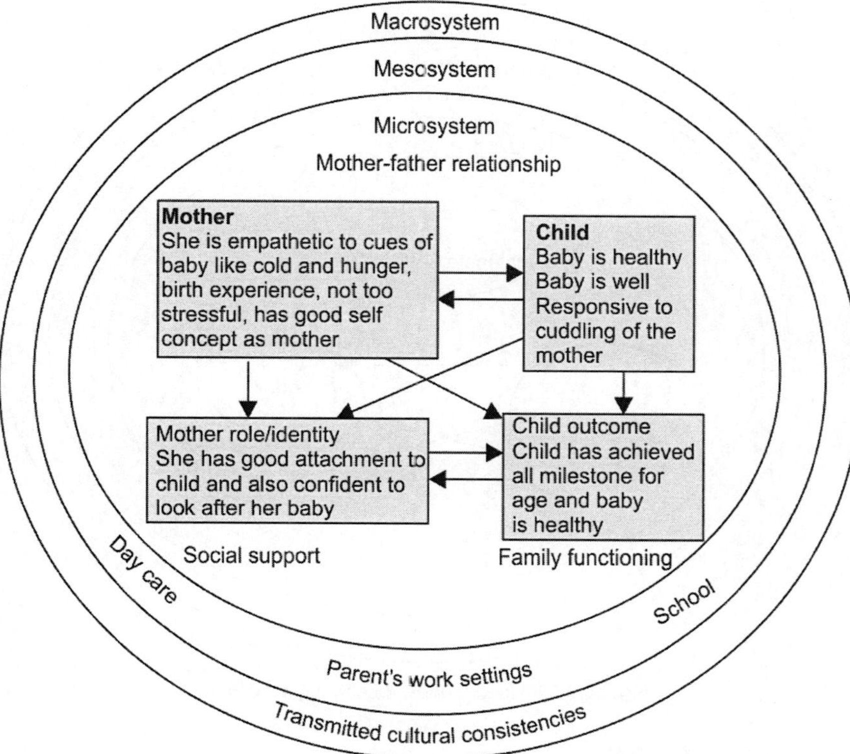

Fig. 28.1: Proposed model of maternal role attaintment

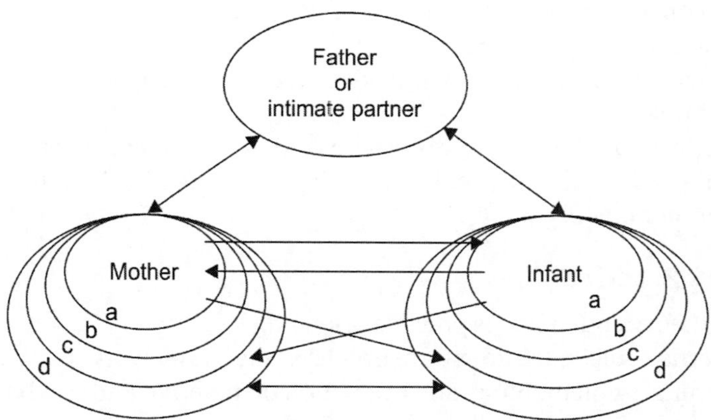

Fig. 28.2: A microsystem within the evolving model of maternal role attaintment

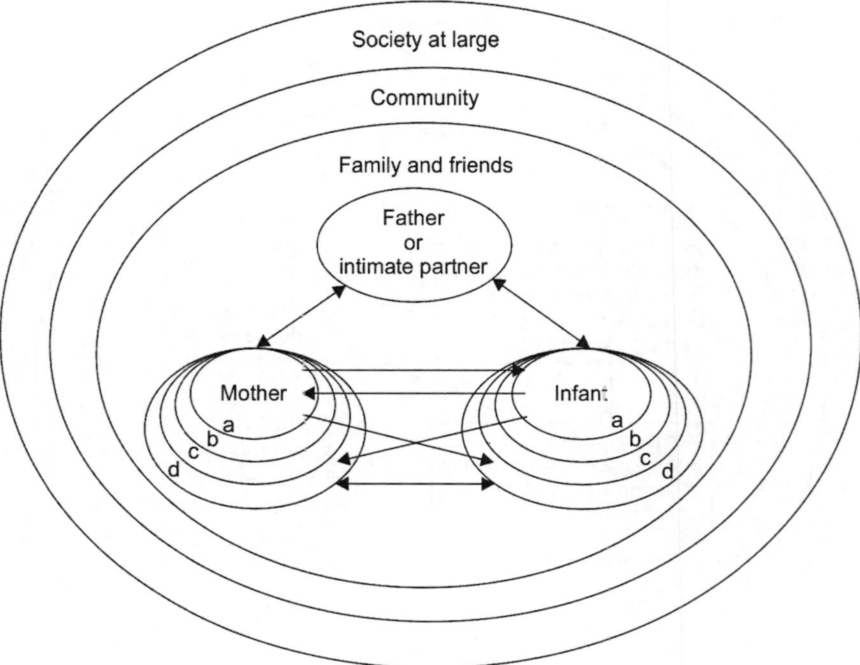

Fig. 28.3: Revised model—becoming a mother

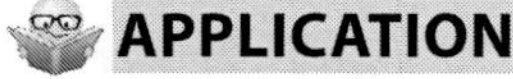

APPLICATION

Nursing Education

- The concepts of Mercer and her model have been used by nursing in numerous obstetrical textbooks.
- The use of Mercer's theory provides a valuable framework for students and nurses.
- An educational program was established for substance abusing women in a residential treatment center based on Mercer's maternal role attainment theory.

Nursing Practice

- Her theory and model is practice oriented.
- Maternal role attainment theory lays the framework for assessing, planning, implementing, and evaluation of maternal and newborn care.

Nursing Research

- Mercer has tested factors that she theorized and/or hypothesized have an impact on maternal attainment. She has reviewed the literature extensively and formulated questions and models that guided researches.
- Mercer's theory is used in graduate student theses and research projects. Also theoretical framework has been used by many in correlation studies and doctoral research dissertations.

Limitations

- Some interchanging of terms and labels used to identify concepts, such as adaptation, attainment; social support and support network are potentially confusing to the learners.
- Concepts are not specific to time and place and are abstract.

CRITIQUE OF THE THEORY

- *Clarity:* The concepts of the theory, variables, and relationships are not explicitly defined but rather are described and implied. They are, however, theoretically defined and operationalized.
- *Simplicity:* In spite of numerous concepts in the theory and relationships, the theory organizes a rather complex phenomenon into an easily understood and useful form.
- *Generality:* This theory is specific to parent-child nursing; can be generalized to all women during pregnancy through the first year of birth, regardless of age, parity, or environment.
- *Empirical precision:* The concepts, assumptions, and relationships are predominantly in empirical observations and are congruent.
- *Derivable consequences:* The theoretical framework for Maternal Role Attainment has proved to be useful, practical, and valuable to nursing. Mercer's work is repeatedly used in research, practice, and education. It is also readily applicable to any discipline that works with mothers and children in the first year of motherhood.

Practical Application of Mercer's Theory of Maternal Role Attainment

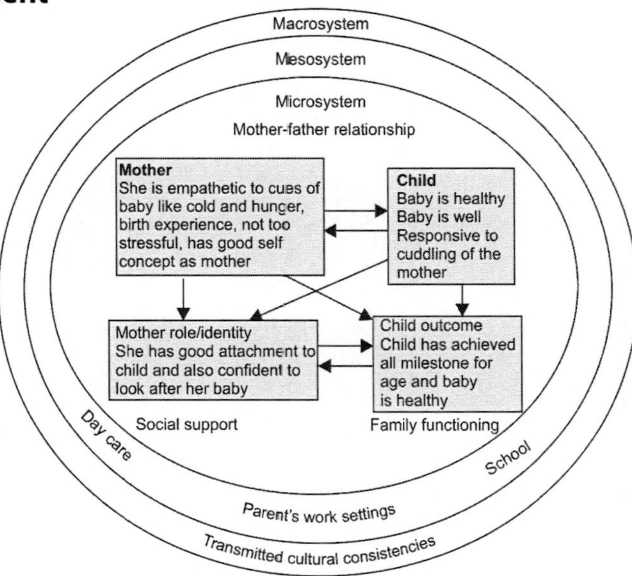

Fig. 28.4: Maternal role attaintment for Mrs Rama

Mrs Rama, 26-year-old delivered a baby boy 9 months before come to immunization OPD for immunization (Fig. 28.4).

CONCLUSION

The Maternal Role Attainment Theory, a mid-range theory, was developed by Ramona T. Mercer to serve as a framework for nurses to provide effective health care interventions for nontraditional women in order for them to successfully adopt a strong maternal identity. Though this theory can be used throughout antenatal period and after childbirth to help women connect with their child, it can also be beneficial for adoptive mothers, foster mothers, or others who have had nontraditional motherhood unexpectedly, such as taking care of a relative or friend's child as the result of a death. The process helps the women form an attachment to hers infant, which in turn helps the child form an attachment with his/her mother. This helps to build the mother-child relationship as the infant grows.

Cornelia M Ruland and Shirley M Moore: End of Life Care

'Standards of care offer a promising approach for the development of middle-range prescriptive theories because of their empirical base in clinical practice and their focus on linkages between interventions and outcomes'.

– Ruland and Moore 1998

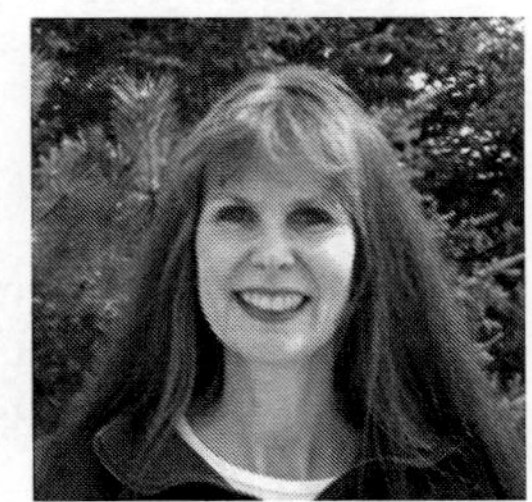

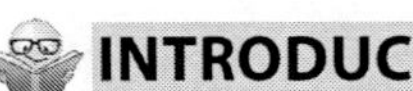

INTRODUCTION

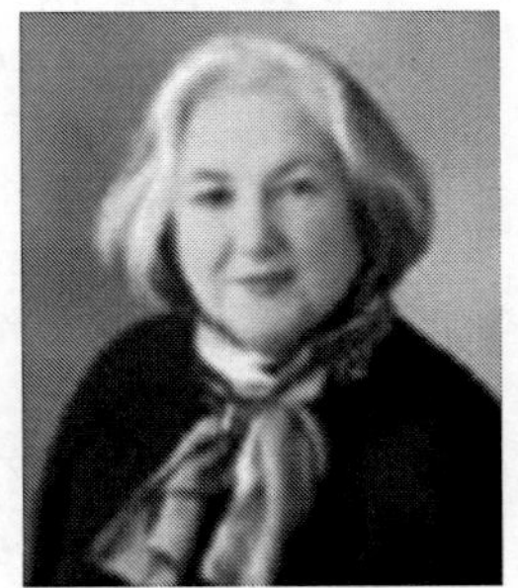

The Peaceful End of Life Theory is a middle-range nursing theory developed by Cornelia M Ruland and Shirley M Moore published in 1998. Peaceful End of Life Theory can adopt everyday nursing practice of terminally ill patients. This theory can be used in all settings of Hospice care, wherever the patient or family chooses such as their home, nursing home, hospital, and in-patient hospice care facility. This theory that help to acquire more knowledgeable about the complex care for the dying patient and how can make it the best experience for the patient, significant other, and family during their peaceful end of life.

Biography and Achievements of Theorists

Cornelia M Ruland

- Ruland began her education at the University of Bergen in Bergen, Norway. Here, she studied undergraduate courses in the field of philosophy and social sciences in 1974.
- She graduated in 1979 with her RN from Haukeland School of Nursing in Bergen.
- She becomes a certified nurse specialist in 1983 from National Hospital in Oslo, Norway with her specialty being in pediatric nursing.
- She obtained her MSN from the University of Oslo in 1994 with an emphasis in nursing administration.
- She received her PhD in Nursing from Case Western Reserve University in Cleveland, Ohio in the year 1998.

- Ruland's nursing career has span over many fields. Her early year as a nurse was focused primarily in the pediatric field.
- She became Assistant Director of Nursing at Aker University Hospital in Oslo, Norway in 1990.
- She has also held the title of Assistant Professor and Adjunct Professor before becoming a Full Professor with the Department of Medicine at the University of Oslo, a position which she still holds today. In May of 2002, Ruland became the Director of the Centre for Shared Decision Making and Nursing Research at Oslo University Hospital, another position she still holds today.

Shirley M Moore

- In 1969 Shirley M Moore received Diploma in Nursing from Youngstown Hospital Association of Nursing.
- She received her BS in Nursing from Kent State University in Kent, Ohio in 1974.
- She received her Master's degree in Psychiatric and Mental Health nursing (1990) and her PhD in Nursing Science (1993) at Case Western Reserve University, Cleveland, Ohio and she worked here as Associate Dean for Research and Professor.
- She has taught nursing theory and science to all levels of nursing students.
- She had leadership roles in professional organizations such as the American Heart Association and Sigma Theta Tau International Honor Society of Nursing.
- Moore also conducts research and theory development in the recovery of cardiac events and has assisted in development and publication in several theories.

Development of the Theory

- The Peaceful End of Life Theory originated as an assignment to derive a middle range theory from a knowledgeable source of the student choice in Doctorial Theory course. This model started when Ruland was a student in one of Moore's classes. Ruland with the help of Moore then developed the Peaceful End of Life Theory from standard of practice made by the Ruland.
- Ruland choose peaceful ending of life as her topic so she just completed a significant project in Norway.
- The development of the peaceful end of life theory included expert nurses on a gastroenterological unit at a hospital in Norway.
- These nurses had a minimum of 5 years, experience with terminally ill patients.
- The study included terminally ill patients, half of whom had been diagnosed with cancer.

- Because there were no clearly defined guidelines to care for the terminally ill, the nurses collaborated to define a standard of care for the peaceful end of life. It also reflected the complexity that is involved with taking care of the terminally ill patient and importance of having knowledge on pain relief and symptom management.
- By developing a theory based on the standards of care set forth by the expert nurses, Ruland was able to provide a base for nurses caring for the terminally ill to follow when caring for patients and their significant others.
- The focus was not on dying in itself but on peaceful and meaningful living during the last days that remained for the patients, significant others, and family members.

 MAJOR CONCEPTS OF END OF LIFE CARE THEORY

The theory is based on the standard of practice for Peaceful End of Life for terminally ill patients. Standard development concentrates on serene and meaningful quality of life in the time that remained patients and their significant others. This standard consists of sixteen outcome criteria. They are the following:

Outcome criteria of the standard of peaceful end of life
The patient • Is not having pain • Does not experience nausea • Does not experience thirst • Experience optimal comfort • Is at peace • Does not die alone **The patient and significant other(s)** • Have confidence that they are receiving the best possible care • Maintain hope and meaningfulness • Participation in decision-making regarding the patient's care • Experience being treated with dignity and respect as a human being • Get assistance in clarifying practical and economical issues related to the Patient's coming to an end of life • Experience a pleasant environment **Significant others** • Are taking part in caring for the patient as they wish • Can say farewell with the patient in compliance with their beliefs, cultural rites, and wishes • Are informed about different funeral procedures and possibilities • Are offered a follow-up visit after patient's death.

It can be discerned that the outcome criteria in the standard were concrete; thus, similar concepts were reduced into summary concepts. They are the following:

Reduction of outcome criteria from the standard to outcome indicators of the proposed theory

Standard	Theory
• The patient is not having pain.	Not being in pain
• The patient does not experience nausea. • The patient does not experience thirst. • The patient does experience optimal comfort. • The patient and significant others experience a pleasant environment.	Experience of comfort
• The patient and significant others participate in decision-making regarding the patient's care. • The patient and significant others experience being treated with dignity and respect as human beings.	Experience of dignity/respect
• The patient and significant others maintain hope and meaningfulness. • The patient and significant others get assistance in clarifying practical and economical issues related to the patient's coming to an end of life. • The patient does not die alone. • The patient is at peace.	Being at peace
Significant others • Are taking part in caring for the patient as they wish • Can say farewell with the patient in compliance with their beliefs, cultural rites, and wishes • Are informed about different funeral procedures and possibilities	Closeness to significant others/persons who care

Five outcome indicators were derived from the sixteen standard outcome criteria that represent the key concepts in this theory. They are:

1. *Not Being in Pain*
   - This concept is defined as not having the experience of pain or free form pain. This is the central part of many patients' end of life experience.
   - Pain is further considered as an unpleasant sensory or emotional experience associated with actual or potential tissue damage.
2. *Experience of Comfort:*
   - The experience of comfort is described 'as relief from discomfort', the state of ease and peaceful contentment, and whatever makes life easy or pleasurable.
3. *Experience of Dignity and Respect*
   - Each terminally ill patient is 'respected and valued as a human being' and having the value of worth. The client being acknowledge and respect as an equal and not being exposed to anything violates the patient's integrity and values.
   - This concept incorporates the idea of personal worth, as expressed by the ethical principle of autonomy or respect for persons, which

states that individuals should be treated as autonomous agents, and persons with diminished autonomy are entitled to protection.

4. *Being at Peace*
   - Being at peace means the feeling of calmness, harmony, and contentment.
   - The individual is free from anxiety, fear, and worry.
5. *Closeness to Significant Others*
   - According to Ruland and Moore, closeness to significant others means 'the feeling of connectedness to other human beings who care'.

Relationships among the concepts of the Peaceful End of Life Theory (Ruland and Moore, 1998). Theory construction based on standards of care: A proposed theory of the peaceful end of life. (*Nursing Outlook*, (46) 4, 174) (*See* Figure on next page).

THEORETICAL ASSERTION OF PEACEFUL END LIFE THEORY

Ruland and Moore identified six relational statements as theoretical assertions for theory as follows:

1. Monitoring and administering pain relief and applying pharmacological or non-pharmacological interventions help the patient to experiences of not being in pain.
2. Preventing, monitoring and relieving physical discomfort, facilitating rest, relaxation and contentment, and preventing complications help the patient to experience of comfort.
3. Including patient and significant others in decision-making regarding patient care, treating the patient with dignity, empathy and respect, and being attentive to the patient's expressed needs, wishes, and preference help the patient to experience of dignity and respect.
4. Providing emotional support, monitoring and meeting the patient's expressed needs for antianxiety medications, inspiring trust, providing the patient and significant others with guidance in practical issue, and providing physical assistance of another caring person if desired help the patient to experience of being at peace.
5. Facilitating participation of significant others in patient care, attending to significant others grief, worries, and questions, and facilitating opportunities for family closeness contribute to the patient's experience of closeness to significant others or person who care.
6. The patient's experience of not being in pain, comfort, dignity and respect, being at peace, closeness to significant others or person who contribute to peaceful end of life.

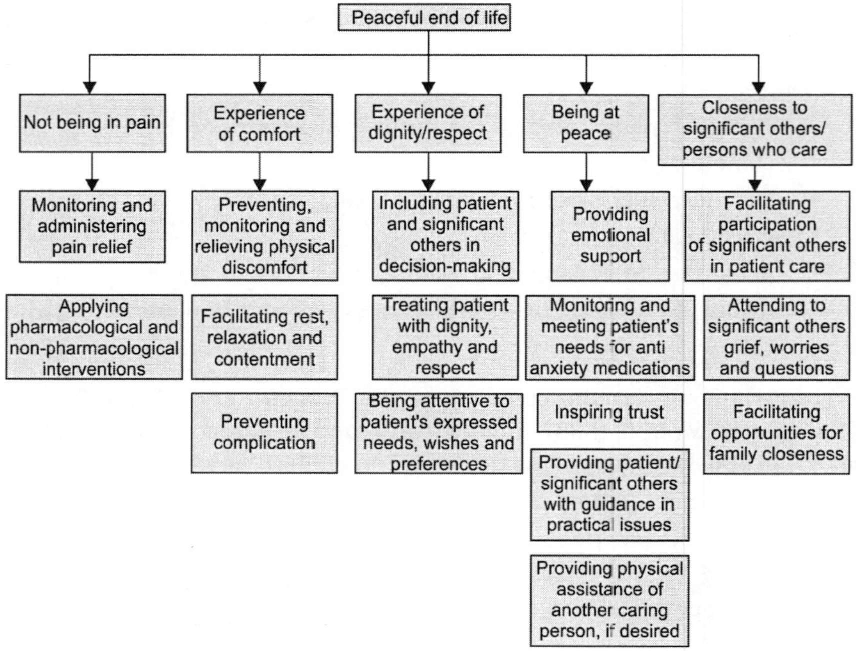

Fig. 29.1: Relationships among the concepts of the peaceful end of life theory

MAJOR ASSUMPTIONS

Nursing, Person, Environment and Health

Ruland and Moore's theory are identified two assumptions as follows:

- The occurrences and feelings of end of life experience are personal and individualized.

  According to them, the one's approach to end of life is a highly personal experience.

- Nursing care is very crucial for creating a peaceful end of life experience. Nurses assess and interpret cues that reflect the person's end of life experience and intervene appropriately to attain and maintain a peaceful experience, even when the dying person cannot communicate verbally.

  Following are two additional, implicit assumptions:

  - *Family:* A term that includes all significant others, is an important part of end of life care.
  - The goal of end of life care is not to optimize care, in the sense that it must be the best, most technologically advanced treatment, a type of care that frequently results in overtreatment. Rather the goal in end of life care is to maximize treatment; that is best possible care will be provided through the judicious use of technology and comfort measures, in order to enhance quality of life and achieve a peaceful death.

APPLICATIONS

Nursing Practice

- By using this theory, nurses are able to give comprehensive care to patients who is terminally ill, significant others, and family with dignity, respect, and empathy.
- It gives guidance to nurses in choosing interventions to decrease suffering and make the last stages of life a meaningful experiences for the patient, significant others.

Nursing Education

- At present, there are no publications that report the use of this theory peaceful end of life.
- This theory can use by students to understand end of life issues.

Nursing Research

- Theory has international recognition as containing key components of a peaceful death.
- Kongsuwan and colleagues (2009) created conceptual model and conducted qualitative and quantitative research on peaceful death in adult patients in Thailand.

Limitations

- The theory is not suitable for all cultures. It is based on Norway culture.
- This theory need more research to back up and to use in nursing research, education, and practice.

Critique

- *Clarity:* Clear in all aspects like in concepts and assumptions. These concepts vary considerably in their level of abstraction, from more concrete (pain and comfort) to more abstract (dignity).
- *Simplicity:* Uncomplicated terms but clear expression of ideas.
- *Generality:* The concept of peaceful end of life is no applicable in all cultures.

PRACTICAL APPLICATION OF END OF LIFE CARE THEORY

Mrs Kiran, 60-year-old widow (one year ago) who was diagnosed with cervical cancer fourth stage. She is mother of five young adult children and grandmother of three. The oncologist ordered home hospice care. She gets care by the nurse and a social worker. She reports high pain level (score 8–10) and difficulty in communication after several weeks of hospice care.

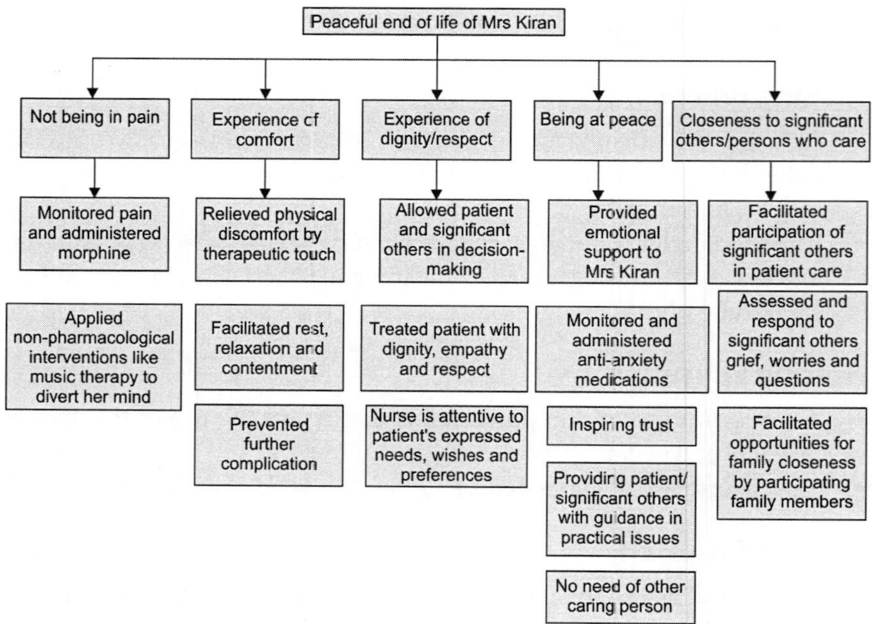

Fig. 29.2: Clinical application of peaceful end of life theory

CONCLUSION

Ruland and Moore developed Peaceful End of Life Care for terminally ill patients who are no longer candidates for curative treatment. The patient and significant others know that death is emanate and this theory provides guidelines on how to physically and emotionally care for, not only the patient but the significant other as well. The guidelines of this theory not only provide standards for peaceful end of life care but they can be applied to all aspects of nursing and patient centered care.

30

Kristen M Swanson: Theory of Caring

'Caring is a nurturing way of relating to a valued other toward whom one feels a personal sense of commitment and responsibility'.

–Kristen M Swanson

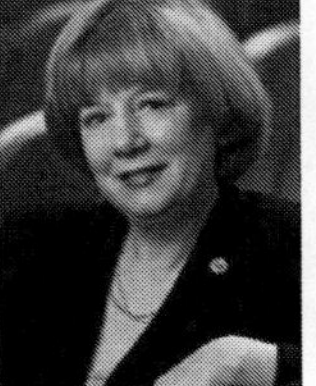

 INTRODUCTION

Swanson's Theory of Caring is based on the research and practice of Kristen M Swanson. Her focus mainly on pregnancy issues. This provides a platform to deal with miscarriage and the subsequent healing required for the parents and family. Kristen M Swanson began her research career studying under Jean Watson, who developed a Theory of Caring. Swanson has modified this theory based upon empirical findings from her research on pregnancy and early fetal loss.

Biography and Achievements

- Kristen M Swanson was born in Providence, Rhode Island on January 13, 1953.
- In 1975, she received her baccalaureate degree from the University of Rhode Island, College of Nursing.
- She earned her Master's degree in nursing (in adult health and illness) in 1978 from the University of Pennsylvania.
- PhD in Nursing program (in Psychosocial Nursing) from University of Colorado in Denver.
- After completion of PhD in nursing science, she received an individually award and National Research Service postdoctoral fellowship from the National Centre for Nursing Research.
- She joined the faculty at the University of Washington School of Nursing.
- She became professor and chairperson of the department of Family Nursing.
- She still conducts research funded by the National Institute of Nursing Research.
- She inducted as a fellow in the American Academy of Nursing in 1991.
- She received alumni award from the University of Rhode Island.

Development of Theory

- During her doctoral student period, as part of hands-on experience with a self-selected health promotion activity, she participated in a cesarean birth support group.
- In one meeting which is focused on miscarriage, she observed that while the speaker, a doctor, who focused on pathophysioloy, and health problems prevalent after miscarriage, women who attended were more focused in talking about their personal experiences with pregnancy loss. She decided to learn more about the human experience and response to miscarriage from that day onwards.
- The main focus became the caring and miscarriage in her doctoral dissertation and her program of research.
- Initial concepts were formulated during her early studies, and as her research progressed Swanson further clarified the five theoretical categories of caring.

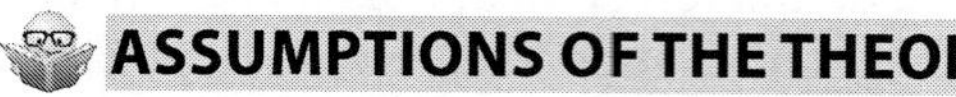

ASSUMPTIONS OF THE THEORY

Nursing, Person, Health, and Environment

- *Nursing and informed caring:* Nursing is an informed caring for the well-being or health of others does not mean that only nurses are caring and she asserts that the nursing discipline is informed by empirical knowledge derived from the humanities, clinical experience and personal and societal values and expectations.
- *Person/clients:* She describes person as unique beings who are in the midst of becoming and whose wholeness is made manifest in thoughts, feeling, and behaviors. The life experiences of each individual are influenced by genetic heritage, spiritual endowment and the capacity to exercise free will. Persons are travel bee and not stagnant.Thus, persons mold and are molded by the environment in which they live in.
- *Health/well-being:* Swanson describes to experience health and well-being is to live the subjective, meaning-filled experience of wholeness. Wholeness involves a sense of integration and becoming wherein all facets of being include many selves that makes us human i.e. our spirituality, thoughts, feelings, intelligence, creativity, relatedness, feminity, masculinity, and sexuality, etc.
- *Environment:* On the basis of situation definition of environment may vary, according to her, for nursing it is any context that influences or is influenced by the designated person/client. She states that there are many influences on the environment, such as the cultural, biophysical, political, social and economic realms, etc. Healing is the process of re-establishing health or well-being, includes releasing inner pain, establishing new meanings, restoring integration and emerging into sense of renewed wholeness.

According to Swanson, the terms environment and person/client in nursing may be interchangeably viewed. For example, 'for heuristic purposes the lens on environment/designated client may be specified to the intra-individual level, wherein the 'client' may be at the cellular level and the environment may be the organs, tissues, or body of which the cell is a component. Therefore, what is considered an environment in one situation may be considered client in another.

THEORY STRUCTURE, CONCEPTS, AND DEFINITIONS

- Swanson proposed five components of caring, i.e. knowing, being with, doing for, enabling, and maintain belief.
- According to her, the proposed structure of the theory depicts caring as 'grounded in maintenance of a basic belief in persons, anchored by knowing the other's reality, conveyed through being with, and enacted through doing for, and enabling.'

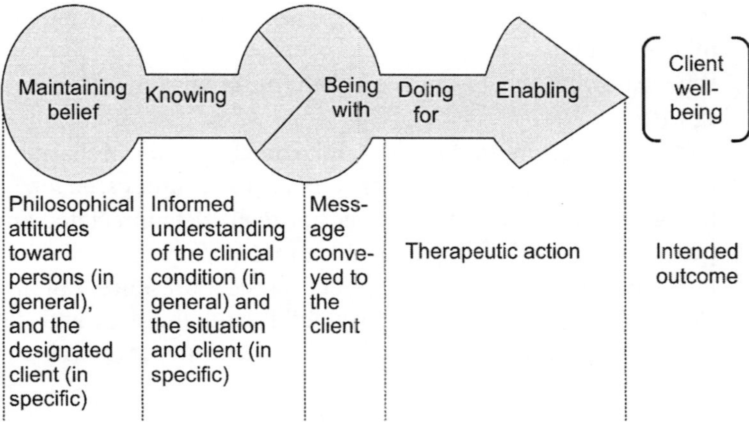

Fig. 30.1: Major concepts of theory of caring

- **Maintaining belief**
  - Sustaining faith or belief in the one's capacity to get through an event or transition and face the future with meaning.
  - Maintaining belief in client is at the base of nursing caring and from this the nurse addresses the care.
  - Caring that maintains belief is the subcategories.
  - Nurses seek to assist clients to attain, maintain or regain meaning in their hospital experience.
  - For example, the nurse is giving care to a mother who is given birth to a stillborn daughter. In this case, the nurse's care centers on monitoring the mother's physical and emotional safety. The nurse build a faith in the mother and through her guidance, will safely and humanely get through the immediate birth and death. Fundamentally, the nurse believes in the family's capacity to create both a dignified passage for

her child and a meaning-filled future for herself: A future wherein her daughter and her birth and death will have a peaceful, permanent meaning in her family's day-to-day existence.

- **Knowing**
  - If maintaining belief is at the base of nursing care, knowing is another factor that moors the belief of nurse.
  - Knowing means striving to understand an event as it has meaning in the life of the other.
  - It translates the idealism of belief maintenance into the realism of the human condition.
  - It involves avoiding assumptions, centering on the one cared for, thoroughly assessing all aspects of the client's condition and reality, and ultimately engaging the self or personhood of the nurse and client in a caring transaction.
  - Subcategories are the nursing interventions.
  - Desire to understand the personal reality of the one being cared for.
  - It helps to recognize the other person as significant and having inherent value.
  - When knowing occurs, both caregiver (nurse) and client are engaged.
- **Being with**
  - It means being emotionally present to other, as a way of sharing in the meanings, feelings, and lived experience of the one-cared for.
  - Being with assures client that his/her reality is appreciated and the nurse is ready and willing to be there for him/her.
  - It includes not just the side-by-side physical presence, but also the clearly conveyed message of availability and ability to endure with the other. For example, call bell in the client room which is a signal for the nurse being there.
  - Presence and sharing are done in such a way that the caring does not burden the client.
  - Being with who goes one small step beyond knowing—it is more than understanding the situation, it is becoming emotionally open to the ones current reality.
  - The message conveyed by being with is that their experience matters to the caregiver (nurse).
  - Sometimes enabling involves substitute care.
- **Doing for**
  - Doing for means 'doing for the other what they would do for themselves if it were at all possible and includes comforting the other, anticipating their needs, performing competently and skillfully, protecting the other from undue harm and ultimately preserving the dignity of the one done for'.
  - It involves actions on the part of the nurse that are that are performed for the recovery of the client.

- **Enabling**
  - Nursing care enables other to practice self-care, and defined as 'facilitating the other's passage through life transitions and unfamiliar events, which includes coaching, informing, and explaining (patient education) to the other; supporting the other and allowing him/her to have his/her experience; assisting the other to focus in on important issues; helping him/her to generate alternatives (thinking it through); guiding him/her to think issues through; offering feedback; and validating (feedback) the other's reality.'
  - Goal of enabling is to assure the long-term well-being of the client.
  - An enabling caregiver is one who uses their expert knowledge to the betterment of the client.
  - Purpose of enabling is to facilitate the client's capacity to grow, heal and practice self- care.
  - Includes providing explanations as well as emotional support by validating the client's feelings.
- **At a glance**

Caring process	Definition	Expressions
Maintaining belief	Sustaining faith in the other's capacity to get through an event or transition and face a future with meaning	• Believing in/holding in esteem • Maintaining a hope-filled attitude • Offering realistic optimism • Going the distance • Helping find meaning.
Knowing	Striving to understand an event as it as meaning in the life of the other.	• Avoiding assumptions • Centering on the one cared-for • Assessing thoroughly • Seeking cues • Engaging the self of both.
Being with	Being emotionally present to the other.	• Being there • Conveying availability • Enduring with • Sharing feelings • Not-burdening.
Doing for	Doing for the other as she/he would do for the self if it were at all possible.	• Comforting • Anticipating • Performing competently/skillfully • Protecting • Preserving dignity.
Enabling	Facilitating the other's passage through life transitions and unfamiliar events.	• Informing/explaining • Supporting/allowing • Focusing • Generating alternatives/thinking it through • Validating/giving feedback.

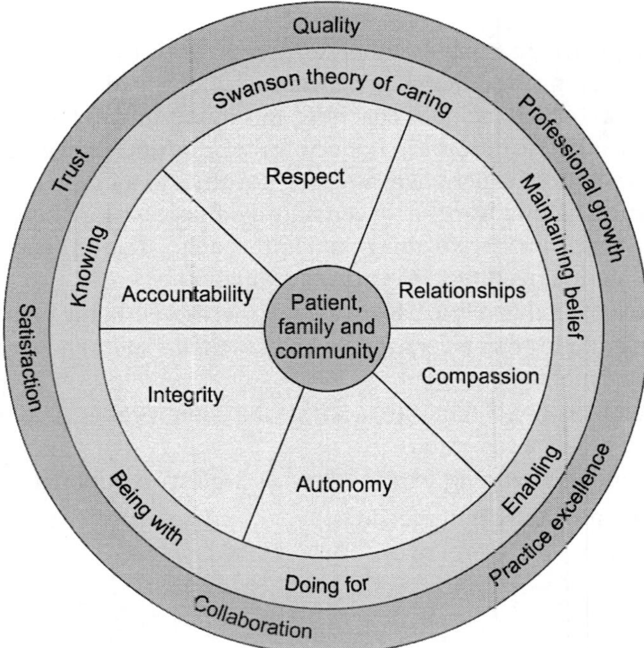

Fig. 30.2: Basic components of Swanson's theory of caring

The theory of caring involves five overlapping processes, best viewed as dimensions of one over-arching phenomenon:

- **Caring**
  - Grounded in maintenance of basic belief in persons
  - Anchored by knowing the other's reality
  - Conveyed through being with
  - Enacted through doing for and enabling others.

APPLICATION

Nursing Practice

- Ahern, Corless, Davis, and Kwong (2011) describe the caring theory application to create advanced practice nursing model of care for anal dysplasia clinic which help to understand the patient's experience, validating feelings, communicating respect, assuring dignity and comfort, fostering a partnership, and creating a positive and self-practice environment to promote the best possible outcomes.
- Andershed and Olsson (2009) conducted a review of research related to Swanson's theory and found that this theory can be applied to many situations like labor room, dementia patients, caregivers of marrow transplantation, etc.

Nursing Education

- By studying the dissertation of Swanson, one can acquire knowledge regarding loss from miscarriage.
- Chokwe and Wright (2012) conducted a study to examine the education process involved with midwives and the application of Swanson's theory of caring was discussed. According to them, 'Swanson's theory is applicable in this study because while socializing the learner midwives into professionalism; a supportive, protective, theoretical-clinical environment must be created such that it enables maintains and cultivates caring, trust and sensitivity'.

Nursing Research

- Andershed and Olssen (2009) conducted a review of research related to studies related to Swanson's theory of caring.
- Dozier, et al. (2001) developed a instrument named the patient perception of hospitalization experience with nursing (PPHEN) which contain 15 point survey assessing patient's perceptions and satisfaction of the care they received while in the hospital. The instrument was developed from Swanson's theory of caring.

Limitation

Unable to study through other methods than phenomenologically.

Critique of the Theory

- *Clarity:* This theory clearly delineates boundaries in each of the five subcategories of caring by identifying, describing, and giving examples of caring behaviors that fulfill each caring process and reducing the risk of ambiguity.
- *Simplicity:* Few concepts and it is easy to understand.
- *Generality:* This theory was originally conceived within a perinatal concept, i.e. miscarriage, but has been successfully applied in many settings: Nursing care including palliative care, dementia, mental disorders, parental support groups, home care, and critical care amongst numerous others, demonstrating a parsimonious theory that boasts a broad diversity of application within the context of nursing practice.
- *Empirical precision:* Swanson's theory of caring is used in many research studies has been found testable and applicable in research. This theory provides a theory based on reality.

CLINICAL APPLICATION OF THE THOERY

Specific Application Scenario by Kari Benton

Sunita is an oncology nurse who is assigned to give care to the Reeja, 20-year-old female with who was admitted with the diagnosis of Acute Lymphocytic

Leukemia (ALL) to her unit. Her family was very supportive and her mother was with her most of the time. She was admitted to the same unit multiple times through a period of about three years for chemotherapy. She was in remission for a time but then relapsed and needed treatment once again. Sunita cares Reeja for many times during her stays until she eventually died of complications of infection.

Knowing

- *Avoiding assumptions:* Sunita build a good relationship with Reeja and because she assumed the best in her and that she was only trying to make sure her daughter was cared for.
- *Centering on the one cared for:* Sunita always spoke directly to her and asked her questions during her assessment daily.
- *Assessing thoroughly:* She cared for Reeja on her first admission to her unit. She continued to care for her for the next three years off and on. Sunita knew from her first experience with Reeja that she was very sensitive to fluid overload. So she always paid very close attention to her fluid status by monitoring her input/outputs and listening to her breath sounds daily.
- *Seeking cues:* Reeja would not always speak up right away when she needed something. But Sunita came to know the certain look in her eyes and change in her behavior when she was feeling uncomfortable. In those instances, Sunita would seek to find the sources of her discomfort.
- *Engaging the self of both the caregiver and the care receiver:* Reeja loved to joke and give people a hard time. She enjoyed when Sunita playfully teased her about always asking her to take so many medications or when it took her a while to return to her room.

Being With

- *Being there:* Sunita often lingered in Reeja's room to have small talk with her and her mother. The times when her mother would leave the hospital for a short time Sunita would check in on her more frequently to make sure that she had everything she needed and she is safe.
- *Conveying availability:* Even if Sunita was not assigned to Reeja, she would always stop in to check on her when she was re-admitted. There was more than one time when as a result of doing that mother was able to share her concerns with Sunita over how her daughter's fluid status was being handled. Sunita was able to speak with the nurse caring for her and let her know about her experience with Reeja and how to prevent her from going into fluid overload.
- *Sharing of feelings:* There was many times Sunita given care to Reeja. There were times her mother cried with Sunita both when her daughter was first diagnosed and later as she relapsed and neared the end of her life.
- *Not-burdening:* Sunita never hesitated to share her feelings for Reeja. She always told her and her mother that she thought she has an extra special

power and a great girl. After her death, she sent a card to the family just showing her appreciation for how well they had raised their daughter and how much she enjoyed taking care of her.

Doing for

- *Comforting:* When Reeja was first diagnosed, she and her mother were very scared and uncertain about the future. Sunita made sure to always explain what was going to happen and answer all of their questions. There were times when Reeja was in pain or uncomfortable and Sunita would not only get her needed medication but would give her a comforting touch as well.
- *Anticipating:* Reeja had difficulty in swallowing pills so she always crushed his medications and gave her favorite drink to take with it. Whenever the doctor's ordered a new medication she made sure to remind the pharmacist that she needed something that was crushable or available in liquid form.
- *Performing competently/skillfully:* Reeja had very sensitive skin and required daily dressing changes on her central line. Everyday made sure to use adhesive remover on her dressing otherwise her skin would be further irritated when removing the dressing.
- *Protecting:* After her experience with Reeja becoming fluid overload very easily, from then on she was her advocate to prevent it from happening again. They had rotated physicians, so not all of them knew her fluids and could not be run faster than 100 mL/hour. Sunita always made sure to get the orders changed so this did not happen, carefully monitored her input/output status. She also made sure to draw her labs first in the afternoon so the results would come back sooner and could start any blood transfusion as early as possible so as to not keep her awake all night.
- *Preserving dignity:* Reeja was very concerned about her privacy when changing or using the bathroom. Sunita always took care to pull the curtain for her or when a Foley's catheter had to be inserted she asked other members to leave the room.

Enabling

- *Informing/explaining:* Especially right after her diagnosis Sunita did so much teaching about the disease and about the chemotherapy drugs she was receiving. Sunita taught them about infection precaution and symptom management.
- *Supporting/allowing:* Reeja went home, she continued to need daily dressing on her central line. Sunita demonstrated the technique to her mother and had her return demonstration and also taught her how to flush her line with saline and heparin.
- *Focusing:* Sunita always tried to let Reeja guide as much of her schedule as possible in order to maintain her self-control. She let her sleep late in the morning and would readjust her medication accordingly. She let her to choose what time she showered and when we did her dressing change.

- *Generating alternatives/thinking it through:* The skin irritation around her central line was probably her most ongoing distress. Together with her mother and with the wound care nurse they created a technique to minimize the irritation. They used adhesive remover, paper tape, and skin preparation. When mother was changing her dressings at home she came up with more strategies for ways to care for the skin that she would share with Sunita the next time she was admitted.
- *Validating/giving feedback:* Reeja and her mother understandably became overwhelmed at times with all that her care involved. Sunita always encouraged Reeja that she was doing such a great job taking all the medications she had to take and letting her to do all the other tasks she had to do. Whenever Sunita would give discharge and always encourage mother that she was capable of managing her care at home. Whenever she raised concerns about her treatment plan she always validated her concerns and made sure to follow up with the doctor. Sunita would tell her multiple times that she knew her daughter better than anyone else, and she should never be afraid to speak up for her.

Maintaining Belief

- *Believing in/holding esteem:* From the time of diagnosis, Sunita tried to educate Reeja and her mother on how to tolerate her treatment as effectively as possible. Sunita assured them that no matter the outcome, they would do everything and could to make Reeja as comfortable as possible.
- *Maintaining a hope-filled attitude:* Sunita rejoiced with them when Reeja went into remission for the first time. When she relapsed, she maintained hope along with them that she could go into remission again, approaching the relapse with as much determination as the first time around.
- *Offering realistic optimism:* Sunita was always straight with Reeja's mother and explained all the risks to her of everything that was being done. Sunita truly did believe in the skill of Reeja's doctor and would share with them her confidence in her treatment plan for Reeja.
- *Going the distance:* Sunita cared for Reeja on and off for about 3 years. She requested to be her nurse or she would visit with her when she was not her patient. When she died, she was on another unit so she heard about it after that. Sunita made sure to send a note to the family to express her sympathy for their loss and her affection for their wonderful daughter.

CONCLUSION

Swanson's Theory of Caring is an exemplar model of a substantive middle-range theory that can 'inform practice and lead to new practice approaches as well as investigate factors that influence the outcomes that are desired in nursing practice'. It delineates five overlapping processes that are best discussed as dimensions of one over-arching phenomenon. For every setting, nursing care is vital part of treatment. So, this theory is very useful for nurses to give comprehensive care to the patient.

Bibliography

1. Alligood MR, Tomey AM. Nursing theory: Utilization and application. 3rd ed. Missouri: Elsevier Mosby Publications; 2002.
2. Carper, BA. Fundamental patterns of knowing in nursing. Adv Nur Sci, 1978; 1(1): 13–23.
3. George, J Nursing theories: The base for professional nursing practice. Norwalk, CT: Appleton & Lange; 2001.
4. Larrabee, JH. Emerging model of quality. Image: the Journal of Nursing Scholarship; 1996;28:353–358.
5. Leininger M. Culture care diversity and universality: A theory of nursing. New York: National League for Nursing Press; 1991.
6. Marilyn E Parker. Nursing theories and nursing practice. 3rd ed. FA Davis.
7. Marriner TA, Raile AM. Nursing theorists and their work. 5th ed. 2005.
8. Meleis Ibrahim Afaf. Theoretical nursing: Development and Progress, 3rd ed. Philadelphia: Lippincott; 1997.
9. Nightingale, F. Notes on nursing: What it is and what it is not. London: Harrison & Sons; 1859.
10. Polit DF, Beck CT. Nursing research: Principles and methods. 7th ed. Philadelphia: Lippincott Williams & Wilkins; 2007.
11. Potter PA, Perry AG. Fundamentals of nursing. 6th ed. St Louis: Elsevier Mosby; 2006.
12. Rosenstoch I. Historical origin of health belief model. Health Educ Monogr; 1974;2:334.
13. Sakraida T, Nola J Pender. The health promotion model. St Louis: Mosby; 2005.
14. Tomey AM, Alligood MR. Nursing theorists and their work. 5th ed. Philadelphia: Mosby; 2002.
15. Wills M Evelyn, McEwen Melanie. Theoretical basis for nursing. Philadelphia: Lippincott Williams & Wilkins; 2002.

Useful websites

- Available from: http://currentnursing.com/nursing_theory/
- Available from: http://nursingtheories.blogspot.in/
- Available from: http://www.nursing-theory.org/
- Available from: http://nursingtheories.weebly.com/
- Available from: http://www.nurses.info/
- Available from: http://nursingtheories-mtctfn2011-2012.blogspot.in/
- Available from: http://nurseslabs.com/

Index

Page numbers followed by *f* indicate figures.

I

J

K

L

M

N

T

V

W